PHILOSOPHY &
PRACTICE
·of Medical Ethics·

© British Medical Association 1988 First printed as 'The Handbook of Medical Ethics' 1984 Second impression 1985 Third impression 1986

Revised as 'Philosophy and Practice of Medical Ethics' 1988

Detailed advice on current issues, including those which may have been altered by legislation, is available from the Secretariat.

British Library Cataloguing in Publication Data:
British Medical Association (Professional Division)

PHILOSOPHY AND PRACTICE OF MEDICAL ETHICS

ISBN 0 7279 0249 0

Published by: British Medical Association, Tavistock Square, London WC1H 9JP

Printed by: Unwin Brothers, The Gresham Press, Surrey. Typeset by: Megaron, Cardiff. In association with Godfrey Lang.

Contents

Preface

Originally, the words 'Ethics' and 'Morals' were Greek and Latin expressions for the same idea – the code of conduct acceptable and normal within a particular society. In the modern world they have come to mean very different things, and it is necessary to stress that this is a handbook of Ethics, not of Morals. The authors believe medical ethics to represent an accepted code of behaviour within a particular group – for our purposes the medical profession – whereas Morals now imply acceptance of a standard outside that group – in the form of a philosophy or a religion.

In reading this Handbook the reader must constantly bear in mind this necessary and implicit distinction between 'Legal' – which is relatively easily determined by reference to statute, 'Ethical' – which is a more difficult assessment of what is currently acceptable and proper to the group of which the reader is a part, and 'Moral' – which requires the reader to view the problem in relation to an authority which the reader accepts personally, even in opposition to other members of the same profession. It is therefore possible, in the judgement of a group, for something to be legal, but unethical, and in the judgement of an individual for something to be ethical but immoral.

We have noted that the word 'Etiquette' has virtually disappeared from current usage in the English language. Nevertheless the concepts of conduct which it described remain. We have therefore deliberately not used this term but replaced it with the term 'Professional Behaviour' which is dealt with in Chapter 8.

The approach to the subject is completely different from that in all previous editions. We have sought to set out the arguments and counterarguments which lead either to universally accepted ethical principles of practice or consensus views. There are some situations in which there is no professional or public consensus and which by their very nature do not permit a consensus view. These require continuing debate and so we have highlighted the current issues in Chapter 15 'Continuing Ethical Dilemmas – No Consensus View'.

This edition of the Handbook of Medical Ethics represents our first major redraft since the 1980 edition was published. We hope the Handbook will serve as an ethical manual so that even if doctors cannot find answers to specific problems, they can work out answers to ethical problems for themselves by applying the principles set out in the Handbook. In addition, from time to time the Association produces updated advice sheets on matters of change. It is our hope that consideration of these issues by the reader will lead him to express his views to the Association.

This book was compiled by the Handbook Working Party, the members of which are as follows:

Dr A J Rowe (Chairman)
Mr K D Fortes-Mayer
Dr J S Horner
Dr A W Macara
Dr S McKechnie
Dr M Wilks

Secretariat

Dr J D Dawson, Head of Professional, Scientific and International Affairs Division
Dr V H Nathanson, Assistant Secretary

Foreword

In 1832 the Provincial Medical and Surgical Association was set up in Worcester. By the time it became the British Medical Association in 1856, a Committee on Medical Ethics had been formed (1849). This Committee was the forerunner of the present Central Ethical Committee (CEC) which is empowered under the BMA's articles and by-laws:

> 'To consider the ethical implications of all matters concerning the relationship between the medical profession, the public and the State, to consider intra-professional ethical matters, to inquire into and adjudicate upon cases involving the professional conduct of any Member, Overseas Associate or Associate Member or any other medical practitioner not being a Member, Overseas Associate or Associate Member with the consent of such practitioner, and to report thereon to the Council and so that the decision of the Committee upon any such case shall be binding upon the parties concerned and upon all Members of the Association and Overseas Associates and Associate Members'.

The Central Ethical Committee has been at the forefront of establishing ethical standards for the medical profession in the UK by contacts with other associations, and by example, the CEC has helped establish norms of conduct for doctors worldwide.

The BMA played an important part in establishing the General Medical Council (GMC) under the Medical Act 1858. The GMC was set up to enable the public to distinguish between qualified and unqualified practitioners; for this reason a Medical Register was created. The GMC was given a regulatory role and found it expedient to issue guidance to all members of the profession from time to time, to enable them to avoid actions which might lead to charges of professional misconduct.

In preparing this guidance, the GMC takes account of the view of the CEC which is also responsible for issuing more detailed guidance on what represents good practice. The publication of guidance by the GMC is in contrast with the practice of other regulatory bodies in some Western European countries, where ethical systems have largely been codified and brought within the national civil and criminal law. In the UK, while a doctor's actions may be lawful, his peers may not consider them ethical.

The GMC's powers derive from the Medical Acts and it is responsible to the Privy Council for enforcing professional standards based on the guidance offered by the profession rather than through a codified system. This means that the UK profession's regulatory mechanism is much more flexible than those of its European counterparts; it can therefore respond rapidly to the changing pressures, expectations and ethics of society and to the medical and ethical questions raised by technological advances.

From time to time the profession reaches an overwhelming view about a particular subject, whether new or not, and debate is unnecessary. This process is sometimes known as prescriptive ethics. At other times, debate is required and the BMA provides a unique forum for this. This is because its democratic machinery allows any doctor to put forward a problem for consideration by the Annual Representative Meeting (ARM) or for advice from the Central Ethical Committee itself. The ARM consists of representatives from all branches of the profession throughout the country and is the largest annual gathering of doctors from all disciplines.

Newly qualified graduates of UK medical schools will have received little or no formal training in medical ethics. Much of the training they have received will have been 'on the job'.

Whether recognised or not, the major influences on the training of UK doctors are Western and Christian. Some doctors may thus experience difficulties in dealing with the various ethnic groups in this country. If this deficiency is not corrected, the problem can only increase, as immigration to the UK has risen since the second world war and particularly since the 1960s.

1 The Background: Philosophical and Religious Influences on the Development of Medical Ethics

Doctors use technical skills and expertise which the untrained person does not possess. Possessing these skills gives him great power over his patients who by the very fact of being patients are dependent, ill and vulnerable. In caring for his patients, a doctor makes a series of judgements and decisions which patients have the right to expect are made fairly in the light of the doctor's knowledge and experience. Most people would agree with these statements.

The argument is about what influences the individual doctor in making judgements and decisions. Professor Ian Kennedy has asserted that the judgements are based not on the doctor's technical skill and training but rather that 'Doctors make decisions as to what ought to be done'. He continued that 'the principles by reference to which we organise our lives and decide what we ought or ought not to do, are not the preserve of any one group'. Nevertheless, he maintained that some believe 'there is a realm of ethics unique to medicine and within the unique competence of doctors to determine and apply. My response is that medical ethics are not separate from but part of the general moral and ethical order by which we live. Decisions as to what the doctor ought to do must therefore be tested against the ethical principles of society'. [Kennedy I. Unmasking Medicine. The Reith Lectures. The Listener, 27 November 1980]

The next question is what constitutes this general moral and ethical order. First of all it is important to recognise that any moral argument is subjective. It cannot necessarily be supported by stringent factual analysis.

The 'general moral and ethical order' is easier to say than to interpret and it is further complicated by the fact that we live in a multi-racial, multi-cultural society. Not only may the 'ethical order' differ within the Christian society but, as will be shown, it is influenced by other religions practised in the United Kingdom. Ethical difficulties may arise when a doctor of one religion or sect, or indeed no religion, is treating a patient with different beliefs and ethical viewpoints.

In western civilisation the obvious place to start when discussing the evolving principles of medical ethics is the Hippocratic Tradition and Oath which date from the 5th century BC. This oath obliges the doctor to '. . . follow that system

1

of regimen which, according to my ability and judgement, I consider for the benefit of my patients, and abstain from whatever is deleterious and mischievous. I will give no deadly medicine to anyone if asked, nor suggest any such counsel; and in like manner I will not give to a woman *a pessary to produce abortion*. With *purity* and with holiness I will pass my life and practise my Art.' Parts of that extract were italicised to illustrate ideas which have been developed by other groups and still strongly influence the judgements of today's doctors, e.g. abortion, professional conduct. The oath was adapted and used by different religious groups – Christians, Jews and Muslims – and was still sworn in this century by doctors in medical schools in Scotland and in Europe.

As a starting point for examining the influences on medical ethics, attention should be paid to the role of the main world religions.

As Jesus told His followers to preach the gospel and heal the sick, there was from the outset a close relationship in Christianity between religion and medicine. Similarly, in Islam there was a duty of care as evidenced by the establishment of Islamic hospitals. The Christian church has a history of promoting care. Care for the sick was institutionalised with the development of Christian hospitals which were based on monastic foundations. When the monasteries were dissolved, England lost not only the shelter and physical care which some provided, but also their records of treatment and pharmacology. The development of medicine from the 17th century required that doctors should develop their own professional identity independent of former religious associations. For a time there was widespread opposition to new medical techniques. More recently there has been a greater readiness to discuss the ethical implications of various kinds of scientific advance; claims to strict autonomy whether scientific, medical or religious have been modified.

The classical Christian approach to general ethical questions has been through the concept of Natural Law which is based on Romans 2:14–15:

> 'When Gentiles who do not possess the law carry out its precepts by the light of nature, then, although they have no law, they are their own law, for they display the effect of the law inscribed on their hearts. Their conscience is called as witness, and their own thoughts argue the case on either side, against them or even for them, . . .'

This in turn has roots in Stoic and Aristotelian ethics.

Using the verses from Romans 2, it is thought possible in the light of reason to discern the laws by which human beings should live in accordance with the given facts of human nature. The Most Reverend J S Habgood, the Archbishop of York, developed this argument as follows:

> 'So far as medicine is concerned, any deliberate interference with normal bodily functioning is, according to this view, a violation of Natural Law, but may be justified on one of two main grounds:

2

(a) the principle of totality, whereby any diseased part of the body may be removed or otherwise modified if its malfunctioning constitutes a serious threat to the whole;

(b) the principle of double-effect, whereby a good action is not forbidden, even if one of its unintended consequences is evil'.

Using such principles, the Roman Catholic Church has developed a detailed set of principles on many ethical issues in medicine. Protestant thinkers have not developed such a systematic approach. This reflects Protestant suspicion of the Natural Law tradition and also the tendency of Reformed Theologians to start from the ethical problems raised in medicine itself rather than abstract principles. Moreover, Protestant theology emphasises Grace to the virtual exclusion of law and so is more amenable to general guidelines concerning Christian attitudes than detailed instructions on behaviour in particular situations. According to Dr Habgood 'many now treat the Bible as a guide to the spirit in which problems must be tackled, an authority for the values which must be preserved, and an exploration of some of the basic issues, such as the ambiguity of human createdness and creativity, which underlie the ethics of scientific advance.'

In common with Christianity, Judaism regards healing as part of man's partnership with God. The governing principle in Jewish medical ethics is the supreme importance of the preservation of life. By this means, things that would otherwise be prohibited in Jewish law are allowed. For example, although it is forbidden to mutilate a corpse, transplants are permitted. Jewish law is against direct use of 'euthanasia' (see Chapter 16 – Continuing Ethical Dilemmas – No Consensus View), but deliberate failure to keep a dying person alive by the use of artificial methods is not viewed so seriously. Reformed Judaism permits all methods of contraception only but Orthodox Jews are permitted to use certain types of contraception if there is a danger to the life of the female from pregnancy. Nowadays, this is usually interpreted more liberally.

Islam's ethical tradition has several foundations. In general, the Arabic world tended to draw from the Greeks in medical science by translating the available texts of Hippocrates, Rufus, Galen, Dioscorides and others. Later there was an attempt to use the Koran to build up an Islamic tradition – 'prophetic medicine'. Several high-ranking Muslims promoted medicine and during the first four or five centuries of Islam, most physicians were Christians and Jews. As a result, the basic ethical text of an Arabic physician was the Hippocratic Oath. Nevertheless, there are some obvious differences between theory and practice. For example, although forbidden in the Hippocratic Oath, abortifacient drugs are often mentioned in the pharmaceutical texts and doctors allowed sterilisation of eunuchs and judicial amputations. The first ethical code would appear to have been put forward under the Ottoman Empire. The reader may wish to refer to the more extensive treatment of this subject in the Dictionary of Medical Ethics (Revised and Enlarged Edition) 1981, published by Darton Longman & Todd, London.

Buddhism is devoted towards purifying the mind with a view to reaching the state of Supreme Enlightenment. The Buddhist emphasis on medical care stems from the idea that physical health is necessary for mental well-being. Buddhists preach that life begins at the moment of conception and should be taken good care of until its end. The end of life is defined as being the death of the body. Any action which causes shortening of life or loss of life is undesirable and should be avoided, e.g. abortion is unacceptable to a strict Buddhist and some countries such as Burma have only recently permitted contraception. It is the duty of Buddhists to provide any help possible for those who need it. Providing sedatives and analgesics in therapeutic doses to relieve physical and mental suffering will make life easier to bear for the sick and those around them. However, giving people too much of these agents so as to cause unnatural loss of life is unacceptable even with the recipient's consent. If the recipient asks for euthanasia, it amounts to suicide, and since self-destruction is a violent act, it is not allowed because Buddhism has a strong peaceful tradition which holds the idea that death should be as natural and peaceful as possible. Buddhists believe that when the body dies, the soul will leave and so the body lacks a spiritual owner and is therefore free to be used by others for any purpose. By this means, Buddhism allows organ donation and tissue transplantation.

The texts upon which Hindu medicine is traditionally founded date from about 700 AD and are attributed to Charika, Susruta and Vagbhata. Physicians were required to be dexterous and learned. They were required to cure or treat but payment of a fee was recognised as a factor in the cure. A physician was not obliged to treat the terminally ill and did not treat a patient who was apparently incurable, hostile to physicians, the king's enemy or an untouchable. Hinduism contains the belief that though many sicknesses are due to the current faults of the patient, many are due to unexpiated sins from previous lives. The physician was protected against suits for damages from a dissatisfied patient but was liable to fines for treating him incompetently, negligently or maliciously. Abortion was regarded as a sin. However, the mother's life was deemed more important than the foetus in cases where a choice was needed. Until the early 19th century, suicide was allowed on various grounds such as being terminally ill provided that the suicide was accomplished in prescribed ways. The physician, however, did not take part in this. Medical experiments were unknown although surgeons could practise on decomposed corpses. Traditional Hindu (Ayurvedic) medicine is still widely practised today alongside western (allopathic) medicine.

Having dealt with the main religious influences on medical ethics, it is necessary to turn to some of the philosophical influences and to examine them critically. Though there are many common themes in all religions, there are differences in emphasis and interpretation which have resulted not only from developments in medical practice and science, but also from the expectations and the more pragmatic attitudes of modern society.

Utilitarianism is probably the easiest philosophical approach to accept and arguably the most difficult to apply. Generally associated with Jeremy Bentham, in crude terms the utilitarian thinker makes a decision which will achieve the greatest good for the greatest number. To take a problem of confidentiality: Do you break confidentiality and tell an unsuspecting foster mother that her husband is the father of the seventeen year old foster daughter's unborn baby? The couple have asked you not to tell and said that they won't, the home is outwardly very stable, the girl intends to leave it anyway as soon as she can. Whose interests are paramount – the foster daughter's, the father's, the mother's or the unborn baby's? The decision of 'greatest good' rests on other factors than the purely moral or legal.

Another approach is based on the absolute right to life of all human beings. This approach includes a veto on killing potential human beings, and the idea that help in life-threatening conditions should not be denied. This concept has obvious religious associations and can be seen in the medical ethical ideas of some of the main world religions. Yet they do not recommend the preservation of life at all costs. It would mean that the highly scientific medicine practised today, which can sometimes maintain a sort of life indefinitely, would try to save every life no matter what the cost or the gravity or the resultant effects of the care that can be provided to other patients. It also raises problems when a patient wishes to die or when a baby will die after a very short period of painful life.

It is universally agreed that a doctor should at least do no harm. This concept is enshrined in the Hippocratic Oath (see earlier) which obliges the doctor to 'prescribe regimens for the good of all my patients according to my ability and my judgement and never do any harm to anyone'. However, doctors may be faced with a choice of harms as in the earlier example of the foster daughter. In such cases the doctor is obliged to judge what is best for the patient in the circumstances of the individual case. This raises questions of 'paternalism' – the assumption that the doctor knows better than anyone, including the patient, what is best for that patient.

Paternalism is in direct conflict with the principle of autonomy. Broadly speaking autonomy means that individuals should have personal liberty to decide their own actions or their own destiny. Although the concept of autonomy is not new it is now becoming a central influence on the expectations of patients. In the past, many patients would accept without question decisions made by their doctor. Today, patients are more critical.

'Truth telling' is another principle by which people address medical ethics. As discussed later in this Handbook, the doctor and the patient are bound by an unspoken, unwritten agreement which is based on the patient's ability to trust his doctor. Truthfulness is therefore seen as important because it is a moral imperative in itself and on utilitarian grounds produces a good social relationship.

5

However, doctors do not always want to tell the patient the truth if the knowledge is likely to cause the patient physical or mental harm. Equally, not all patients tell the whole truth to their doctors. Nevertheless, patients' expectations in this area have led to most doctors increasingly telling patients more about their condition and the possible or probable outcome.

Doctors have been accused of protecting their own. Where malpractice or incompetence come to light, doctors face a difficult personal decision over what to tell the affected patient, the appropriate professional body responsible for this or, ultimately, the employing or legal authority. The profession's duty is to the patient; its honour can only be maintained by acceptance of that duty.

While medicine is in some respect an exact science, physically and mentally the human race is infinitely variable. To communicate with a patient, often distressed, is an art which doctors should develop. At its peril does the medical profession forget the kindness and reassurance of the 'bedside manner'.

The influences on medical ethics have only been addressed superficially in this chapter. However, it should already be clear that principles conflict and cannot be applied absolutely. Religion does not always help either. So what is left? Although faulty, the principles and religions are not in themselves wrong. They provide a framework which a doctor may use to make decisions. The argument was summed up very neatly by Dr Habgood who, in commenting on the history of medical ethics for this edition, said:

> 'It seems to me that one of the clearest lessons to be learnt from the history of medical ethics is that most of the interesting and difficult problems have no logical answers. This is not to say that ethical thinking need be unprincipled or reduced to mere expressions of opinion, but simply that the real dilemmas arise when facts are ambiguous, prognostications hazardous and principles are in conflict. A good moralist is one who has learnt to live with this uncomfortable mixture and weigh the significance of the various factors involved'.

and, as Dr J P Horder suggested to the working party revising this Handbook:

> '. . . if well established rules based on evidence and experience were missing . . . the need for decision and action made one invent rules of a sort. Otherwise there was just a pathless desert. One could not afford the uncertainties of the philosopher'.

2 The Social Contract: Autonomy and Paternalism

The Doctor/Patient Relationship

Together, the 1944 Education Act and the 1946 National Health Service Act, in the context of an unprecedented period of peace and a developing social security structure have revolutionised public attitudes and expectations. Universal free education to university standard and comprehensive health care have in general made people better informed, more conscious of their potential rights and more capable of expressing their expectations. On the other hand, the increasing complexity of high technology medicine often involves greater risks as well as greater benefits. Patients, by reason of their illness, are vulnerable and it cannot be assumed that the individual patient in a given situation necessarily understands the possibilities and problems which it presents.

A successful doctor/patient relationship is most important in providing effective health care. The form this relationship takes will vary according to the patient's needs and attitudes. The doctor should take his lead from the patient and adapt his approach to each consultation or relationship after following the indications given by the patient. He should not forget that the patient has come to him for help and advice. The doctor should try to deserve and win the patient's trust and confidence. Equally he should learn to trust and understand patients' judgements about themselves. In this way, the two parties develop a complex set of understandings which form an unwritten contract between them.

In the past the doctor/patient relationship tended to rely heavily upon a paternalistic approach by the doctor. Originally such an approach arose because of the inequality of knowledge between them. The doctor, as the expert, used his superior knowledge and made decisions on health care issues which many people could not hope to comprehend. Over many years, this has led to the development of a medical mystique and thus a failure to communicate. This attitude cannot continue in the face of developments in general education and the advent of the modern media of mass communication. Increasingly patients have begun expressing a desire to know what is wrong with them and to understand the action taken by their doctors. Many wish to

7

participate in decision-making. This attitude began to emerge strongly after the second world war and has been particularly noticeable since about 1970. It is only in the past three or four decades that the full significance for medical practice of the philosophy expounded by the 18th century philosophers, John Locke, J-J Rousseau and Kant began to be fully appreciated. We are now experiencing a change from paternalism into partnership. Simultaneously, more emphasis is being placed on the patients assuming responsibility for their own health, especially concerning the effects of their own way of life on their health.

The World Medical Association's (WMA) International Code of Medical Ethics, adopted in 1947, began to reflect this move from paternalism to partnership. The WMA followed this initiative by adopting ethical codes and statements on a number of related subjects such as: Human Experimentation – The Declaration of Helsinki 1964; Rights of the Patient – The Declaration of Lisbon 1981; Therapeutic Abortion – Declaration of Oslo etc. These are reproduced at the end.

In the US, groups including the American Hospital Association have set out statements of patients' rights which are based on principles such as autonomy and veracity. These American codes differ from earlier codes as they focus on the rights of those receiving health services rather than on the obligations of health professionals. This reflects the historical and mental characteristics of a nation founded and fed by successive waves of emigrants fleeing persecution in their native land. It also reflects a system in which most of the working population pay directly for each item of health care. US government agencies have reflected this trend by action in public policy e.g. in 1974 Congress created the National Commission for the Protection of Human Subjects of Biomedical and Behavioural Research. The Commission's conclusions, raise questions about the proper relationship between the government and the profession.

In Europe, and in particular within the European Community, similar trends can be seen. These initiatives largely stem from the consumer groups and have resulted in Parliamentary questions, debates and resolutions in the European Parliament on such subjects as a Charter of Patients' Rights, the Rights of Children in Hospital etc. These Community initiatives reflect in varying degrees activities within the Member States themselves, as well as those of international consumer groups.

In the UK the evolution of a 'partnership approach' has been reflected in the development of the Patients' Association, the Community Health Councils and bodies such as the College of Health.

Doctors must recognise the value of this 'consumerist approach' to medicine. They should always be aware of their ability to choose to be paternal if that is what their patient needs or to choose to involve the patient as far as the patient requires. Doctors will inevitably face instances where one type of behaviour is more appropriate and effective than the other. It is necessary to maintain a flexible attitude particularly as the patient's needs may vary during consultations and treatment. Patients do not merely wish to have their own views taken into account but to have things explained in a manner which they can understand and to share in decisions which affect themselves far more than they affect the doctor.

In practice, three types of professional relationship exist between a doctor and a member of the public:

(i) The first and most common form of relationship is the therapeutic doctor/patient relationship. This is where a person consults a doctor seeking professional advice and skills about a medical problem affecting him. Using the principles explored in this Handbook the doctor employs his professional knowledge to advise the patient. The implied contract requires that the doctor will use his skills to the best of his ability not only to treat the condition which is the subject of the consultation but also, when appropriate, to advise how best the patient should conduct himself in order to maintain his health. The doctor is responsible to the patient for his actions. In this form of relationship, the doctor should act only in the best interest of the patient.

(ii) In the second form of relationship the doctor acts as an impartial medical examiner and reports to a third party, e.g. in relation to a pre-employment medical or insurance. Such examinations are often made by the doctor who normally has a therapeutic relationship with the patient. The information gathered by that doctor will be used for purposes other than the health care of the patient. In these circumstances, the doctor is being asked to act in a different role. The nature of this role must be clearly explained to the patient as the patient must be in a position to make a decision as to whether to give consent to the disclosure of the information the doctor holds about him.

Equally, reports requested by a third party with the consent of the patient may be prepared by a doctor who has no previous professional relationship with the patient. In such circumstances, the patient may properly wish to limit the information he shares with the doctor. The doctor can only report on the basis of information presented to him. The doctor has a duty to explain the nature of the relationship to the patient before proceeding with the examination.

If a report is requested by a third party with the patient's consent, the patient should generally be given the opportunity of seeing the report and indicating whether it should be sent. If the doctor decides that it is not in the patient's interest to see the report, he should be prepared to justify this. Any decision by a doctor to send a report against the patient's wishes would have to be justified in terms of the overriding public interest.

Issues of consent are discussed in Chapters 3 and 4.

(iii)   In the third form of relationship the doctor engages in clinical or other research in the interests of the advancement of medical science, in the interest of a group of people or even in a personal line of enquiry. As in (ii) above, the doctor should be scrupulous in explaining the nature of his role in relation to the patient particularly if he normally has a therapeutic relationship with the patient.

Research is discussed in chapter 14.

The Patient's Choice and the Management of Health Care

A person is free to choose the doctor from whom he wishes to obtain medical advice. Equally, a doctor is free to accept or refuse anyone as a patient, subject to the constraints of his professional and contractual obligations, such as:

(a)   In an emergency where a doctor is bound to provide any treatment immediately necessary and to ensure that arrangements are made for any further treatment.

(b)   In isolated communities where the doctor is the only source of medical advice.

The organisation and rules of Social Security may have the effect of limiting the choice of those patients participating in the scheme. In NHS general practice, a Family Practitioner Committee has the power to assign a patient to a doctor whether the doctor agrees or not. This mechanism is designed to ensure that the rights of 'difficult' patients under the NHS are not diminished. If a doctor conforming with the procedure laid down in his terms of service removes a patient from his NHS list he should inform the patient why.

Patients and prospective patients need to be able to obtain factual information about the range of services available. For this reason, general practitioners are encouraged to issue practice information booklets designed to enable the public to choose the service which best suits their needs. These booklets should be low key, factual and should not draw attention to achievements, educational or otherwise, of the doctors or the practice as a whole. In no circumstances should they be 'self-promotional' an activity which is contrary to the guidance given by the General Medical Council and which continues to be deprecated.

It is good medical practice in the UK for one doctor to be responsible for the overall management of a patient's illness. This system helps to ensure that a patient with a particular complaint is assessed as a whole. Furthermore, following a series of such encounters, a doctor/patient relationship is gradually built up with benefits to both. If trust exists between them, the patient will feel more confident and happy with the service which the doctor provides. Furthermore, the doctor will acquire the basic personal health information about his patient, some or all of which may be relevant in treating any particular illness. This knowledge held by the primary doctor is an important factor in the considerations that follow.

A patient is free to approach a doctor other than his usual one. If the patient is not under active treatment by his usual doctor, any doctor is free to accept him as a patient, although this doctor should consult the patient's usual doctor in accordance with good medical practice. Such consultations must have the patient's consent.

However, if a patient is already under treatment but chooses to consult another doctor, he must accept that normally the doctor will refuse to treat him unless he terminates the previous clinical relationship. If this course is adopted the patient should inform his previous doctor that he is receiving care from another doctor.

Except in an emergency a doctor in whatever form of practice should take positive steps to satisfy himself that a patient who applies for treatment or advice is not already under the active care of another doctor before he accepts him. Not only is this in the patient's interest but it is also in the doctor's. If the patient is under active treatment he should be told why his usual doctor should be contacted before medical care begins. If the patient does not consent to this procedure, the doctor may refuse to treat him unless the patient is prepared to terminate the previous clinical relationship. The doctor should also, where possible (see below), notify the original doctor.

A patient may request a second opinion about a particular illness. Such requests should be handled sensitively by the patient's usual doctor and the patient should not be made to feel a 'nuisance' or a 'bad patient'. The patient may well have reasons for requesting a second opinion which he does not feel able to share with his usual doctor. A request for a second opinion can sometimes reflect a failure in the doctor/patient relationship or a failure in communication. The doctor should attempt to assess objectively whether this is the case and, if so, whether anything can be done to rectify it.

Having taken account of the principles set out above where a doctor agrees to undertake the care of the patient, he must accept the responsibility of ensuring continuity of care of the patient.

The Importance of Communication

Good communication between doctor and patient is the foundation of a good relationship which will ensure optimal use of the doctor's professional knowledge and skills and also the patient's understanding and co-operation.

It is vital to be able to explain problems to patients orally, using terms which are well understood and at the same time avoiding over-simplification. Usually it is unnecessary to limit what patients are told but rather to explain problems they may have. Such communication protects the patient from unnecessary alarm. In cases where alarm is justified good communication can offer comfort and reassurance. Time spent on communication is time well spent. The ability to listen is a fundamental skill; some patients need to feel that their doctor is their friend and should not feel rushed in outlining their problems to the doctor. Equally, tact is required when dealing with the patient's relatives.

In certain circumstances a doctor may not always be able to follow those recommendations because of language difficulties. In such cases the patient, his relatives, or the doctor should try to find someone who can act as translator.

Communication skills are essential to the practice of medicine. Patients expect to receive information about their condition. Unless there are compelling reasons to the contrary this expectation should be fulfilled. This may include allowing patients access to their medical records [see: subject access, Chapter 3]. If, for some reason, the doctor feels unable on clinical grounds to divulge information requested by the patient, he should be prepared to justify the decision. Care and sympathy are needed in explaining the decision to the patient.

Rapid and clear communication between professional colleagues engaged in the care of a patient is essential. If continuity of care is to be properly maintained, essential information must be available to the physician who becomes responsible for that patient's immediate continuing care. This applies, for example, where a patient under treatment by his medical practitioner moves to another area, or when a patient enters or is discharged from hospital. It is vital that a preliminary discharge letter is sent; and it must be clearly legible. The doctor from whose immediate care the patient is passing should decide the best means of communication, having regard to the circumstances and the likely delay in receiving a posted letter. The use of abbreviations should be avoided wherever possible; they may lead to misunderstanding.

The practice of medicine also increasingly requires frequent communication with other professions. The physician has at all times a 'duty of clarity'. Whether engaged in discussion in the multi-disciplinary forum, telephoning instructions to a ward, or writing a prescription or other therapeutic note, the doctor should aim to eliminate ambiguity, doubt or illegibility. Clear messages diminish the possibility of mistakes and harm to patients.

Referral

As stated earlier, the practice of medicine is based on the concept of one doctor, the general practitioner, taking charge of the overall management of a patient's health care. Clearly this doctor cannot have the specialised skills to treat every condition presented by a patient any more than a specialist would have all the skills of a general practitioner. The general practitioner therefore has a responsibility to obtain information about appropriate specialist services and, if necessary, refer a patient. As co-ordinator, the general practitioner is able to build up a record of referrals and draw inferences which may not otherwise have been apparent. Letters of referral to a colleague and requests for specialist diagnostic investigations should therefore refer to any aspects of the patient's history which, though not immediately relevant to the subject of referral, might be important in any action by the specialist.

Referral to Another Medical Practitioner

The method of referral from a general practitioner to a consultant or specialist has evolved in the patient's interest. The GMC, in its booklet, 'Professional Conduct and Discipline: Fitness to Practise (April 1987)', states:

'ACCEPTANCE OF PATIENTS BY SPECIALISTS

Although an individual patient is free to seek to consult any doctor, the Council wishes to affirm its view that, in the interests of the generality of patients, a specialist should not usually accept a patient without reference from the patient's general practitioner. If a specialist does decide to accept a patient without such reference, the specialist has the duty immediately to inform the general practitioner of his findings and recommendations before embarking on treatment except in emergency, unless the patient expressly withholds consent or has no general practitioner. In such cases the specialist must be responsible for the patient's subsequent care until another doctor has agreed to take over that responsibility.

In expressing this view the Council recognises and accepts that in some areas of practice specialist and hospital clinics customarily accept patients referred by sources other than their general practitioners. In these circumstances the specialist still has the duty to keep the general practitioner informed'.

A doctor in consultant or specialist practice should not accept a patient without reference from a general practitioner except in the following circumstances:

(a) In an emergency.

(b) If he is asked for a confirmatory opinion or specialist opinion on a different aspect of the case by the specialist to whom the patient has been properly referred.

(c) If reference back to the general practitioner would produce delay seriously detrimental to the patient. The specialist should inform the general practitioner as soon as possible of the action he has taken and the reasons for it.

(d) If referred by doctors in the school or other community child services – but only after the general practitioner has been given the opportunity to refer the child himself.

(e) If it is for a consultation in sexually transmitted disease.

(f) If enquiry indicates that the consultation is for a refraction examination only.

13

(g) If a patient is formally referred by a physician from outside the United Kingdom.

(h) If the patient is seeking contraceptive advice and treatment and is unwilling to consult her own general practitioner about contraception, or she states that her own general practitioner does not provide contraceptive services. At the time the advice and treatment is sought it should be explained to the patient that it is in her own best interests that her general practitioner be informed that contraception has been prescribed and of any medical condition discovered which requires investigation or treatment. Every attempt should be made to obtain permission to contact the general practitioner before prescription or fitting of a contraceptive device. This is particularly important if the patient is at the same time under the active clinical care of her own general practitioner or that of another doctor.

(i) If the patient is seeking therapeutic abortion and is unwilling to consult her own general practitioner or, having done so, is unable to secure his agreement to refer her to another doctor. It should be explained to the patient that it is in her own best interest that her general practitioner be informed of the treatment or advice given. Every attempt should be made to obtain the patient's permission for this.

A medical practitioner may have special skills; he may use acupuncture or hypnosis as part of his treatment. The use of these skills in relation to a patient for whom he is not the usual medical practitioner is practice analogous to that of a specialist. If he accepts a patient without reference from a general practitioner other than in the circumstances outlined, he must observe the GMC guidance set out above.

Referral to Specialists who are not Medically Qualified

In recent years nurses, physiotherapists, psychologists and other health care professionals have increasingly performed specialised health care functions upon delegation from a doctor. This trend is welcome. There is also a growing demand by patients for referral to practitioners of complementary medicine, e.g. osteopathy, acupuncture. The patient's right to choose complementary medicine should be respected provided the patient behaves responsibly. In all such cases the referring doctor must be satisfied that those to whom he is delegating specific tasks have the knowledge and skill required to perform them. In the case of practitioners without professional registration this entails some form of personal vetting. Doctors should consider the following extract from the GMC booklet Professional Conduct and Discipline: Fitness to Practise (April 1987):

'The Council recognises and welcomes the growing contribution made to health care by nurses and other persons who have been trained to perform

14

specialised functions, and it has no desire either to restrain the delegation to such persons of treatment or procedures falling within the proper scope of their skills or to hamper the training of medical and other health students. But a doctor who delegates treatment or other procedures must be satisfied that the person to whom they are delegated is competent to carry them out. It is also important that the doctor should retain ultimate responsibility for the management of his patients because only the doctor has received the necessary training to undertake this responsibility.

For these reasons a doctor who improperly delegates to a person who is not a registered medical practitioner functions requiring the knowledge and skill of a medical practitioner is liable to disciplinary proceedings. Accordingly the Council has in the past proceeded against those doctors who employed assistants who were not medically qualified to conduct their practices. It has also proceeded against doctors who by signing certificates or prescriptions or in other ways have enabled persons who were not registered medical practitioners to treat patients as though they were so registered'.

It is important that a doctor should not reject a patient who has consulted, without referral, an alternative practitioner. The doctor should still treat the patient and counsel him about why a referral by a general practitioner might have been more appropriate.

Referral for Private Health Care

The principles involved in referring a patient for private health care are no different from any other sort of health care. However, patients are vulnerable in medical matters by reason of illness and lack of expertise. It is therefore unethical to charge them excessively for a service, to persuade them to accept a service which they do not need, or persuade them to receive that service in circumstances where the benefit is to the doctor and not to the patient. The doctor is under the obligation at all times to give advice and treatment which are clearly in the patient's best interest.

If a doctor has a financial interest in a private facility of such a size that it is strongly to his personal advantage to persuade patients to use the facility in preference to equally suitable alternatives, he places himself seriously at risk of a charge of unethical conduct. He must be particularly scrupulous about disclosing that interest.

If a doctor's financial interest in a private facility is on such a modest scale that it indicates professional commitment rather than personal advantage and that facility is of such a high standard that its use raises no ethical issues, it may be considered unnecessary to lay any requirement upon the doctor to disclose that interest. Nevertheless, attention is drawn to the GMC guidance on this subject from the GMC Booklet 'Professional Conduct and Discipline: Fitness to Practise (1987)', Paragraphs 105 and 106:

'A doctor who recommends that a patient should attend at, or be admitted to, any private hospital, nursing home or similar institution, whether for treatment by the doctor himself or by another person, must do so only in such a way as will best serve, and will be seen best to serve, the medical interests of the patient. Doctors should therefore avoid accepting any financial or other inducement from such an institution which might compromise, or be regarded by others as likely to compromise, the independent exercise of their professional judgment. Where a doctor has a financial interest in an organisation to which he proposes to refer a patient for admission or treatment, whether by reason of a capital investment or a remunerative position, he should always disclose that he has such an interest before making the referral.

The seeking or acceptance by a doctor from such an institution of any inducement for the referral of patients to the institution, such as free or subsidised consulting premises or secretarial assistance, may be regarded as improper. Similarly the offering of such inducements to colleagues may be regarded as improper'.

The Doctor/Patient Relationship in Law

Ethical and legal responsibilities are closely related. Though the ethical code does not, in this country, form a branch of the law, there are a number of occasions when the ethical practice and the legal 'standard of care' are inseparable.

Before the National Insurance Act 1911 and the National Health Service Act 1946, medical law in England was dominated by the contractual relationship of doctor and patient. Apart from a number of specific statutory duties, such as the reporting of certain infectious diseases, doctors and surgeons tended to provide their services under direct contract to the patient or occasionally to a benevolent society. The legal thinking which developed around the practice of medicine was largely derived from the law of contract. The Act of 1946 greatly modified this contractual relationship.

The National Health Service Acts consolidated in the Act of 1977 charge the Secretary of State with the overall responsibility to provide hospital, medical, and other allied services. Modern medical law is complex for many reasons: the operation of the necessary supporting administrative structure; the changes brought by frequent parliamentary interventions; and the flow of circulars from the Health Departments.

The complexity has not in any way diminished the 'legal standard' of patient care. The doctor's responsibility for standards of medical care has been defined by the GMC in its booklet Professional Conduct and Discipline: Fitness to Practise (April 1987)' as follows:

16

'The public are entitled to expect that a registered medical practitioner will afford and maintain a good standard of medical care. This includes:

(a) conscientious assessment of the history, symptoms and signs of a patient's condition;

(b) sufficiently thorough professional attention, examination and, where necessary, diagnostic investigation;

(c) competent and considerate professional management;

(d) appropriate and prompt action upon evidence suggesting the existence of a condition requiring urgent medical intervention; and

(e) readiness, where the circumstances so warrant, to consult appropriate professional colleagues.

A comparable standard of practice is to be expected from medical practitioners whose contribution to a patient's care is indirect, for example those in laboratory and radiological specialties'.

The doctor's position in NHS practice, however, cannot be considered in isolation from his contractual obligations to the employing authority or Family Practitioner Committee.

The right to carry on medical practice is closely regulated under the Medical Acts 1858 to 1983. Until 1969 the General Medical Council had the power to erase from the Register the name of any fully or provisionally registered practitioner judged by the Disciplinary Committee of the Council to have been guilty of 'infamous conduct in a professional respect'. Undoubtedly such a finding would have included a failure to conform to the ethical standards of the profession. Since the Medical Act 1969, these powers are related to the phrase 'serious professional misconduct' which replaces the previous phrase 'infamous conduct in a professional respect'.

3 Confidentiality

The principle of confidentiality is basic to the practice of medicine and fundamental to the doctor/patient relationship. It was contained in early codes such as the Hippocratic Oath:

> 'Whatever, in connection with my professional practice, or not in connection with it, I see or hear, in the life of men, which ought not to be spoken of abroad, I will not divulge, as reckoning that all such should be kept secret'.

Patients attend their doctor in the belief that the information they supply to the doctor or which the doctor finds out about them in the course of investigation or treatment will be kept secret. This encourages them to speak frankly and thus provide the doctor with clues or information which can be essential to diagnosis or treatment. The patient must be able to feel certain that going to the doctor will not result in an outcome which will have an undesirable effect on this life, e.g. gossip about having a particular disease etc. This has a desirable result for society as a whole; people with communicable diseases are not deterred from seeking treatment for fear of the consequences.

Although confidentiality is a long-accepted principle, confusion arises among doctors in understanding the principle and in applying it. Largely this can be resolved by examining the reasons for confidentiality. As stated above, the patient is concerned that by consulting a doctor his autonomy and privacy could be threatened.

In the UK, medical information is not privileged in law. This was expressed clearly by Lord Denning as Master of the Rolls in the case of Attorney General v Mulholland and Foster [1 All E.R. 767].

> 'The only profession that I know which is given a privilege from disclosing information to a Court of law is the legal profession and then it is not the privilege of the lawyer but of his client. Take the clergyman, the banker or the medical man. None of these is entitled to refuse to answer when directed to by a judge. Let me not be mistaken. The judge will respect the confidences which each member of these honourable professions receives in the course of it, and will not direct him to answer

unless not only is it relevant but also it is a proper and, indeed, necessary question in the course of justice to be put and answered. A judge is the person entrusted, on behalf of the community, to weigh these conflicting interests – to weigh on the one hand the respect due to confidence in the profession and on the other hand, the ultimate interest of the community in justice being done'.

The doctor tries to protect his patient's interest in respect of confidentiality. If the patient's claim to confidentiality were not accepted doctors would be reluctant to record information, as would be the patient to confide in him. If confidentiality is broken by a doctor then the onus in UK civil law is on the patient to seek compensation using arguments in relation to the consequences of the doctor's action. There is also recourse to the GMC's Professional Conduct Committee but the Committee is unable to award any financial recompense to the patient. In some other Western European countries, however, the doctor who breaks confidentiality may be punished under both the criminal and civil law as well as by his registration authority.

It can be argued that the doctor also has reasons for wishing to preserve confidentiality. These are in relation to the judgements and decisions he makes as an expert. Some doctors fear that if medical information were to be shared widely, clinical decisions might be questioned. This is seen by some as a threat to the doctor's clinical autonomy and his position in society. These feelings are a natural result of insecurity and doctors must try to overcome them. If not, defensive medicine could ensue and the patient's interests would not necessarily be served.

Despite the doctor's interests in maintaining confidentiality it must be agreed that the crucial reasons for maintaining it relate entirely to the patient's interests, not those of the doctor.

In applying the principle, further difficulties arise. The principle is not always easy to defend and conflicts increasingly occur with the greater participation in health care by some professions who do not have ethical codes, e.g. in multi-disciplinary teams. Extended confidentiality works in respect of doctors' sharing of *necessary* information with medically qualified colleagues, because doctors should all be applying the same principles and are responsible to the GMC for their professional conduct. However, the doctor sharing information with someone not bound by an equally stringent code is making a disclosure of information for which he is responsible.

In trying to set out guidelines to help doctors make decisions on confidentiality the BMA has been accused of making principles and exceptions so wide as to be meaningless. Nevertheless, we believe that the following guidance gives a basis for practical reasoning.

1. The doctor is responsible to the patient with whom he is in a professional relationship for the confidentiality and security of any information which he obtains.

2.   A doctor must preserve secrecy on all he knows. The fundamental principle is that he must not use or disclose any confidential information which he obtains in the course of his professional work for any purpose other than the clinical care of the patient to whom it relates. The following are the only exceptions to this principle:

 (i) If the patient consents;

 (ii) If it is in the patient's own interest that information should be disclosed, but it is either impossible, or medically undesirable in the patient's own interest, to seek his consent;

 (iii) If the law requires (and does not merely permit) the doctor to disclose the information;

 (iv) If the doctor has an overriding duty to society to disclose the information;

 (v) If the doctor agrees that disclosure is necessary to safeguard national security;

 (vi) If the disclosure is necessary to prevent a serious risk to public health;

 (vii) In certain circumstances, for the purposes of medical research.

The doctor must be able to justify his decision to disclose information without consent. In making such a decision, he should always remember that he may, at any time, be required to justify it. When he is in any doubt about a particular course of action he should consult the head office of the BMA or his defence body.

Consent to disclosure

The information that a doctor obtains about a patient remains the property of the patient. However, the patient may, in certain circumstances, authorise the doctor to share it. A patient's general authority may be assumed for the necessary sharing of information with other professionals concerned with his health care, both for any particular episode and, where essential, for his continuing care. However, beyond this the patient's express consent must be obtained before any disclosure is made. This consent is valid only if the patient fully understands the nature and consequences of the disclosure. In such cases the doctor, in seeking consent, should make every effort to explain to the patient the implications of disclosing information, and the extent of the proposed disclosure. If consent is given, the doctor is then responsible for limiting the disclosure to the extent to which the patient has consented. In obtaining consent the doctor should not burden the patient with unnecessary information which may alarm the patient unduly.

Information shared with other doctors or members of other health professions may be given in the normal form of a clinical report. In all other cases it must be given in the form of a report appropriate to the particular circumstances.

21

Disclosure in the patient's own interest

Confidential information may need to be disclosed to a person having a close personal relationship with the patient, in order that that person can help him to manage his condition. Normally, the patient's consent should be sought for such disclosures. However, the patient's condition may itself preclude him from understanding what is involved, or there may be special circumstances which render it medically undesirable in the patient's own interest for him to be told the full implications of his condition. In such circumstances, the doctor may in his discretion disclose information without the patient's consent to a relative or other appropriate person, to the extent necessary for the patient's own interest, having regard to the particular circumstances of the case.

There is however a particular problem which doctors may encounter upon which the ARM has repeatedly given clear guidance. This concerns certificates of illnesses suffered by a deceased patient in the period immediately prior to taking out a life insurance. These certificates, known as 'Duration Certificates', are unacceptable to the Profession, which encapsulated its view in the resolution passed in 1962 and reaffirmed in 1964 and 1983:

> 'That this Meeting strongly recommends practitioners not to issue 'duration certificates' (i.e. certificates to insurance companies re. the medical history of a person who had died soon after acceptance – without report – for life assurance)'.

Disclosure required by law

A doctor may be required by law to disclose confidential information without the patient's consent either because:

1. An Act of Parliament (or a regulation made under it) says that he must disclose it in some given circumstances; or

2. An Act of Parliament (or a regulation made under it) has empowered someone else to say that he must disclose it for some given purpose; or

3. A Court of Law has made an order for disclosure in a particular case.

Professional discipline over all such disclosures is exercised by the GMC, within guidelines issued from time to time. A doctor is always free to follow his conscience in refusing to disclose information even if the law requires him to, provided he is ready to take the consequences which the law imposes [Hunter v Mann 1974]. Such a refusal although illegal may not necessarily be unethical. If the doctor is in any doubt as to what to do in a particular case, he may obtain advice from his local BMA liaison officer, BMA Head Office, or his medical defence body.

Court Orders

In the UK there is no legal privilege for communications between patient and doctor; a Court can therefore compel a doctor to give evidence, and direct him to disclose confidential information when giving it. A refusal to comply with such a direction could constitute a contempt of Court, punishable by fine or imprisonment. When asked by a Court to disclose information without a patient's consent, the doctor should first refuse on the grounds of professional confidence, and explain why he feels that the disclosure should not be made. The Court will normally take such a statement into consideration, but if it nonetheless orders the doctor to answer the questions, he will have to decide as a matter of conscience whether he should comply.

A Court may also order the disclosure of medical records before a trial at which evidence is given in civil claims based on personal injury or death. The law concerning this is contained in sections 33 to 34 of the Supreme Court Act 1981. Broadly, these empower the Court to order the disclosure of medical records to:

1. A person who is an actual or potential litigant; or

2. His legal adviser; or, if the applicant has no legal adviser;

3. A medical adviser nominated by him; or

4. A combination of 1 and 2.

The Court has a discretion to decide which of these methods is to be used, and any doctor who is in doubt as to the most suitable procedure in any case is advised to consult his medical defence body.

Doctors who are approached by solicitors for access to their records are recommended to seek advice from the BMA or their defence body, as the law on this subject is now very complicated.

Overriding duty to society

Unless an Act of Parliament or a Court order specifically requires it, a doctor is under no legal obligation to disclose any confidential information without the patient's consent. However, like every other citizen, a doctor has moral responsibilities as a member of society. Occasions may arise which persuade the doctor that confidential information acquired in the course of his professional work should be disclosed. In such cases, the doctor should wherever possible seek to persuade the patient to disclose the information himself, or to consent to the doctor's disclosing it. Failing this, it will be for the doctor to decide on his next course of action in accordance with his conscience, bearing in mind that he may be called to justify what he does.

In the course of their professional work, doctors will often receive requests from the police for access to personal medical information. When considering the balance between the public interest and his duty to the individual patient, the doctor should start from the premise that information obtained by him about a patient in the course of a professional relationship must be kept secret. There may well be occasions when the public interest will clearly outweigh the doctor's duty to an individual patient – for instance where the enquiries relate to a crime so grave that the safety of the doctor's other patients, or of the public at large, is at risk. On other occasions the balance may be finely drawn. The doctor must be aware that if, after the most careful consideration, he decides to disclose to the police information which he has obtained in confidence, he may later be called upon to justify his action, either before the GMC or in a Court. Before a doctor decides to make such a disclosure, he should satisfy himself:

1. About the gravity of the crime concerned;

2. That the prevention or detection of the crime will be seriously prejudiced or delayed if the information is not disclosed; and

3. That the information will not be used for any other purpose, and will be destroyed if no prosecution is brought, or if it does not lead to a conviction.

Doctors who have difficulty in reaching a decision, having considered the facts presented to them by the police, are advised to discuss such requests with the BMA, or their defence body.

National Security

In exceptional cases, a doctor may be asked to disclose information to a member of the police Special Branch or of the security services, in order to safeguard national security. Here again, other than the Prevention of Terrorism Act 1984 which is currently operative only in Northern Ireland there is no law which requires him to do so, but he may well feel obliged to agree to the request as part of his moral responsibility as a citizen. Before he does so he should satisfy himself that the enquiry is one which does affect national security, and that the disclosure is necessary to safeguard security. If he is shown a certificate to this effect personally signed by a Cabinet Minister, the Attorney General, or the Lord Advocate, he may treat this as sufficient evidence.

Public Health

Under public health legislation a doctor is legally required to notify certain diseases and conditions to the appropriate authorities. However, a doctor may sometimes think it right to make disclosure beyond the legal requirement, where he considers it necessary to prevent serious risks to public health, for example in the prevention and control of communicable diseases, or through the monitoring of adverse reactions to drugs. If the doctor intends to make such a disclosure, he should first satisfy himself that the information will not be used for any other purpose.

Medical Research

Research into health and disease may benefit existing or future patients, or lead to improvements in public health generally. Such research often requires access to confidential personal health information about identified patients. Normally, such information should not be used or disclosed for research without the patient's consent. However, this may not always be practicable in the case of some kinds of research; also, it could in some cases be against the patient's own interest to ask him for it.

In these circumstances, the information should only be used or disclosed only if a local ethical research committee has satisfied itself that a sufficient case has been made for dispensing with the patient's consent and has approved the research proposal. Among the conditions which such a committee will normally impose will be:

1. That the researchers will secure the data adequately against unauthorised access, and will not disclose them to anyone outside their team;

2. That no patient will be identifiable from any published results; and

3. That all the data will be destroyed when they are no longer required for the research.

If the doctor is approached by researchers for information about his patients from his records, he should not disclose it unless he has either obtained the patient's consent, or he has satisfied himself that an appropriate ethical committee has approved the research, and had dispensed with the need for consent. Even then, he must not disclose information about any patients if he is aware that they object to such disclosure.

If researchers ask the doctor for permission to approach his patients direct, the doctor must first satisfy himself that the research has been approved by an appropriate ethical committee, and then give his permission only if he is satisfied that the patient will not suffer any adverse consequences from such an approach. Normally, he should seek the patient's consent before he gives permission.

If the doctor is himself involved in the research, he is responsible for ensuring that the approval of an appropriate ethical committee is obtained before the research begins, and that all conditions imposed by the committee are strictly complied with.

Teaching

Clearly in order to carry out undergraduate and postgraduate clinical teaching, personal information about a patient has to be shared from time to time with the students. It is important that the patient's informed consent should be obtained for teaching to take place and also that the students understand the nature and importance of confidentiality and its preservation.

Security of storage and access

The doctor must ensure, as far as he can, that all medical information is kept in a secure place.

The following statements apply to record systems in all disciplines of medical practice, and set out the basic criteria for access to records which include clinical information:

(a) In all medical records, information should be regarded as held for the specific purpose of the continuing care of the patient, and should not be used, without the consent of the patient or appropriate authorisation by the responsible clinician, for any other purpose.

(b) Access to identifiable information held in medical records should be restricted to the author and the person clinically responsible for the patient during the episode for which the data were collected (or their successors), unless specifically authorised by the clinician in the interests of the patient. Access to clinical data of previous episodes of illness should be available to the clinicians currently providing care for the patient.

(c) Where records containing identifiable personal data relating to the physical or mental health of any person are held on a computer maintained by a health authority, the use and disclosure of such data will be regulated by the DHSS Code on Confidentiality of Personal Health Data. Doctors should help health authorities to comply with this Code, and should apply it wherever possible to their own records, whether or not these are computerised.

(d) Home office regulations will be made under section 2 of the Data Protection Act 1984.

(e) Tribunals service committee enquiries etc may have statutory rights to obtain information. This too is detailed in the DHSS Code on Confidentiality.

If a doctor has doubts about the security or confidentiality of his patients' records in any records storage system, he should refuse to place clinical information in them.

Subject Access (Patient Access to Records)

In the 1987 session Parliament passed a Bill relating to the access by individuals to records containing personal information about them. This does not extend to access by the subject to his own medical records. There has been in recent years an increasing movement towards openness between the doctor and his patient which is referred to elsewhere in the Handbook. Part of the profession considers that patients should have the full right of access to their personal medical records. The profession is much divided on this issue.

The concern to avoid any harm to the patient from direct access to the records is summarised in the statement of the Inter Professional Working Group (IPWG) on Access to Personal Health Information (Appendix I).

The General Medical Services Committee of the BMA has issued advice to GPs on the practical procedures ensuing from a subject access request. This is attached as Appendix I.

A further important consideration is that many records contain information about third parties; this also is privileged information which would require the third party's permission for its disclosure to the subject of the personal medical record or any other person.

There has been much public and professional debate on this issue following the Data Protection Act 1984, its recognition of the patients' right of access to automated information held about them on their behalf and the current Bill which is an extension of this debate into the field of manual records.

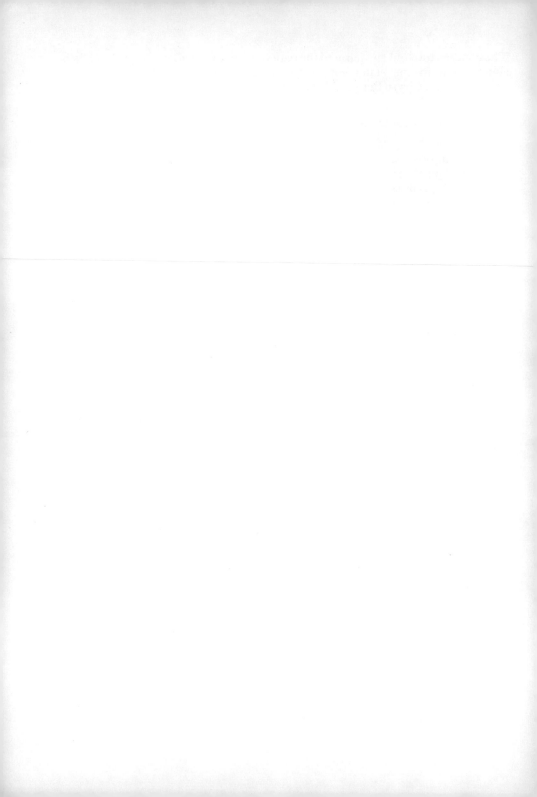

4 Consent to Treatment

The basis of any discussion about consent is that a patient gives consent before any investigation and treatment proposed by the doctor. Doctors offer advice, but the patient decides whether to accept it.

Before a patient can consent, the options have to be presented in such a fashion as to allow a decision to be made. Consent must involve the ability to choose. One of the patient's options is not to be troubled with having to make a decision. Doctors sometimes argue that patients do not want to be told all the facts. In an increasingly articulate society doctors are moving away from this paternalistic approach and any doctor who decides to withhold information should examine stringently the reasons for doing so. Society is moving away from paternalism towards partnership and at the same time people are taking increasing responsibility for the effects of their own way of life including its effects on health. Even though a few patients 'don't want to be told', there is now little justification for withholding information – unless 'to tell all' would be clearly detrimental to the individual. It is therefore only when the patient specifically delegates responsibility for the decision to the doctor that it is ethically right for the doctor not to disclose all the relevant facts.

Normally, the patient will wish to decide. The doctor should remember that his specialised training and knowledge puts him in a powerful position compared with the patient who will usually lack the detailed knowledge to grasp the essential facts immediately. The lack of this knowledge does not mean that the patient is unable to understand. Consent without understanding is invalid and it is the doctor's moral, professional and legal duty to help the patient reach this understanding. In so doing the doctor should follow the patient's lead and present as many of the risks and benefits as the patient needs to know.* Naturally a doctor can only discuss matters in relation to the accepted state of medical knowledge at the time.

One of the problems about consent is that it must follow disclosure of information and thus understanding of the medical condition. As UK case law

---

*The doctor would be well advised to have regard to patients in whom levels of consciousness are impaired, post head injury states and impaired consciousness due to intoxication.

has evolved, the amount of information that a doctor is legally obliged to disclose to a patient in the context of consent to treatment is based on the concept of what information a reasonable member of the medical profession would give the patient in a particular set of circumstances to enable him to reach a decision. This has been most recently affirmed by the 1983 Sidaway case [1985, 1 A11 E.R. 643] which explored the concept 'informed consent'. Equally, cases and allegations about lack of consent are usually based on assault and battery or negligence. It is important to remember that a doctor's legal obligations are much less than his moral obligations. The legal minimum is not necessarily ethical.

Exceptions

While the principles of consent remain, there are exceptions in particular situations. These are emergencies, and the treatment of minors, the mentally incompetent and the senile.

Despite recent legal cases, no legal minimum age has been set for consent to treatment. It has been suggested that sixteen is the 'Age', as section 8(1) of the Family Law Reform Act 1969 states that 'the consent of a minor who has attained the age of sixteen years to any surgical, medical or dental treatment which, in the absence of consent, would constitute a trespass to his person shall be as effective as it would be if he were of full age: and where a minor has by virtue of this section given effective consent to any treatment, it shall not be necessary to obtain any consent for it from his parent or guardian'.

However, the Act goes on to state that 'nothing in this section shall be construed as making ineffective any consent which would have been effective if this section had not been enacted'. As the Common Law position before 1969 was uncertain, there remains in effect no set minimum age for consent.

Thus the criterion for consent should not be age but competence. This is an entirely subjective judgement based upon the individual child and the circumstances when the child presents. Little difficulty is raised where a patient under the age of sixteen requires immediate treatment when no parent or guardian is available. Emergencies cannot wait for consent and there can be little doubt that a court, having regard to parents' duty to provide medical care for their child, will uphold the doctor's action in providing such care as might reasonably anticipate the parents' consent. If there is difficulty in contacting the parents, the doctor must assess the urgency of the need for treatment before embarking on any procedure.

Similarly, if the treatment is minor, such as for a cough or cold, the doctor is not likely to be faced with a difficult judgement in relation to an under sixteen's ability to consent. If treatment is difficult, dangerous or raises moral issues, the doctor may experience difficulties including external pressure placed upon him by society's perception of the situation. The most contentious issues relate to advising and providing treatment on contraception and the termination of pregnancy.

Opinions have been expressed that doctors providing contraception, even with the parents' consent, for minors under the age of sixteen might be aiding and abetting the offence of unlawful sexual intercourse. Legal advice is that if the doctor acts in good faith in protecting the girl against the potentially harmful effects of intercourse, he would not be acting unlawfully. Furthermore, Lord Scarman stated in the House of Lords' judgement in the case of Gillick versus West Norfolk and Wisbech Area Health Authority and the Department of Health and Social Security [1985, 3 A11 E.R. 402] that:

> 'If the prescription is the bona fide exercise of his clinical judgement as to what is best for his patient's health, he has nothing to fear from the criminal law or from any public policy based on the criminality of a man having sexual intercourse with her'.

If a girl under the age of 16 requests contraception but refuses to allow her parents to be informed the question of the validity of the girl's consent is raised. It appears that section 8(3) of the Family Law Reform Act 1969 would consider such consent valid in certain cases.

When faced with this problem, a doctor should take the following steps:

(a) Attempt to convince the girl of the advisability of involving her parents in this decision. This should be part of the counselling extended over a number of interviews, where appropriate. In many cases the doctor will gain consent to involve a parent or a person in loco parentis.

(b) If he is unsuccessful, the doctor must then decide whether the girl has the mental maturity to understand his advice and the possible consequences of her action. If she has not, then her consent is not informed and so invalid. The doctor cannot provide treatment in these circumstances but should keep confidential the fact and content of the consultation.

(c) If he is satisfied that she can consent, he makes a clinical decision as to whether the provision of contraception is in the best interests of the patient.

(d) A decision not to prescribe does not absolve him from keeping the interview confidential.

Lord Fraser of Tullybelton, in the House of Lords' judgement October 1985, in the case of Gillick versus West Norfolk and Wisbech Area Health Authority and the Department of Health and Social Security, expressed the following line of conduct for a doctor in such a situation:

1. That the girl (although under sixteen years of age) will understand his advice;

2. That he cannot persuade her to inform the parents that she is seeking contraceptive advice;

3. That she is very likely to begin or to continue having sexual intercourse with or without contraceptive treatment;

4. That unless she receives contraceptive advice or treatment her physical or mental health or both are likely to suffer;

5. That her best interests require him to give her contraceptive advice, treatment or both without the parental consent.

Mental Health

When an adult is mentally incapable of giving valid consent, e.g. by reason of mental illness, serious subnormality or senility, the doctor must decide, as in any other case, what is in the best interests of the patient. No other individual, unless duly appointed as a guardian, has legal authority to consent to treatment on the patient's behalf. The doctor's authority in these matters depends however on the type of treatment and his own status under the 1983 Mental Health Act.

Exceptionally, the doctor may also consider any threat posed to others by the patient's condition. Any doctor who is clinically in charge of a patient at the relevant time may initiate or participate in compulsory admission to hospital for treatment, but the fact of admission to hospital under a section of the Mental Health Act does not necessarily indicate the patient's ability to give or withhold consent. The patient's right to give or withhold consent to treatment for a physical condition is not lessened by the fact of his being admitted under such an Act. What must be considered is whether the patient is able to appreciate the reasons for the nature of, and the possible consequences of, the proposed treatment, and what would happen if the proposed treatment were withheld.

In the mentally handicapped child under the age of eighteen sterilisations should be performed only after the courts have granted wardship. Other procedures – such as minor non-emergency surgery – may be consented to by the parent or guardian.

In the mentally handicapped adult recent court cases appear to imply that no-one, not even the courts, can give valid consent on the patient's behalf. (Reference, Re: B (A Minor) (Sterilisation), reported in 'The Times' Law Report, 1 May 1987). In these cases the courts may rule that the medical intervention will not act against the best interests of the individual.

The legal complexities lead to enormous practical difficulties and consideration is being given by groups such as MENCAP for the need for clarification of the laws.

Detained Persons

In the case of police surgeons, consent carries a number of aspects. A detained person will, in general and by nature of being confined and/or intoxicated, be less free to give consent. He may also be restricted in terms of privacy during the consultation. Under all circumstances, with the exception of intimate body searches, a person in custody is not obliged to submit to medical treatment. The same right applies in the provision of specimens for forensic examination, and the person should be so informed. In the case of an unconscious prisoner, and where ability to give valid consent is inhibited by intoxication, examination and procedures to ensure proper medical care are appropriate; the taking of specimens for forensic purposes is not. These matters are dealt with in chapter 5.

Police surgeons are reminded that special circumstances exist regarding consent to intimate body searches; they are invited to consult the BMA guidelines on this (Appendix II).

Consent to Operations on Reproductive Organs

The other main problem concerns the reproductive systems.

The custom of obtaining the consent of the patient's spouse to operations on the reproductive organs is one of courtesy not legal necessity. Nevertheless, because the patient's partner may properly hold that he or she has an interest in such an operation, it is good practice to attempt to get both partners' consent. Similar considerations apply to the investigation or treatment of the foetus or embryo, or of the intra-uterine environment, particularly as the foetus cannot give any consent.

The limited 'rights' of the unborn child derive from the Offences Against the Person Act 1861 and the Infant Life Preservation Act 1929. The Abortion Act 1967 on the other hand, by legalising the termination of pregnancy within certain limits, diminishes the protection which an unborn child otherwise had. Doctors should have regard for these considerations when the mother refuses treatment for the foetus.

Abortion, and the ethical problems associated is referred to in more detail in chapter 15.

Obtaining consent

At times consent is implied, as in attendance for an inoculation which implies that the patient expects the inoculation. This does not, however, absolve the doctor from explaining any risks. Equally there are times when oral consent is not sufficient and written consent essential. It is important that consent should be free of any form of pressure or coercion, particularly where treatment is offered to patients such as those serving in the Armed Forces, in other types of employment which limit the individual's freedom of action, and to prisoners serving a custodial sentence. No influence should be exerted through any special relationship between a doctor and the person whose consent is sought. This matter is discussed more fully in chapter 5.

The GMC has said of the relationship between doctors and their patients:

> 'Patients grant doctors privileged access to their homes and confidences. . . . Good medical practice depends upon the maintenance of trust between doctors and patients and their families, and the understanding by both that proper professional relationships will be strictly observed. In this situation doctors must exercise great care and discretion in order not to damage this crucial relationship'.

The doctor/patient relationship is based on trust. The doctor will be constantly on his guard to be objective in his judgement in the face of the many outside pressures which may be exerted on him. These may be economic pressures from relatives, advertising, the media, or from other sources.

A doctor is entitled to decline to provide any treatment which he believes to be wrong, but there is a distinction between treatment which a doctor believes to be detrimental to a patient's best interests and treatment to which a doctor has a conscientious objection. A doctor must not allow his decision as to what is in the patient's best interest to be influenced by his own personal beliefs. If a person who is already a doctor's patient requests treatment which the doctor believes to be against the patient's best interests, he should tell the patient and point out that the patient has the right to seek advice elsewhere. If a person who is found by the doctor to need treatment which the doctor cannot provide or take part in because of the doctor's own principles, the doctor must tell the patient and ensure that the patient is referred to alternative medical care.

5 The Doctor and the State

Modern medical practice necessarily brings the doctor into contact with the State in which he practises. Some doctors may be employed to provide medical services on behalf of a State; in other less common cases the doctor's ability to provide care may be seriously compromised by restrictions imposed on his patient's liberty by a State. It is these latter cases which must first be considered since it cannot automatically be assumed that a State's actions are always benign. When the doctor is no longer able to provide completely independent medical care he has an ethical duty to ensure that the patient is aware of the full implications of the doctor's reduced role. In addition, the doctor must always be watchful to ensure that any erosion of independence is identified at the earliest possible opportunity.

The doctor has a first duty to treat and care for an individual patient. He also has a wider duty to serve humanity as a whole. The State has no place in the doctor's loyalty and service in his role as a physician. As a citizen of the State, the doctor has responsibilities towards it. As a doctor he may be remunerated for using his skills for certain groups or individuals within the State, but he cannot as a doctor subordinate his conscience to the State because his responsibilities towards humanity transcend the confines of national interest.

The State's involvement in the doctor/patient relationship may in some cases lead to the assumption of wider powers over individual freedom. This is an insidious development; by the time that ethical issues have become clear and unmistakable to all, the opportunity to curtail the power of the State may already be dangerously weakened. It is therefore essential that doctors concerned about developments within their own individual professional practice should bring them to the attention of the profession as a whole even if no action is ultimately considered to be necessary. Similarly, the profession as a whole must take action at an early stage, firstly because the individual doctors themselves are less likely to be compromised by their involvement in the procedure under question. Secondly, the State apparatus is likely to be more vulnerable to effective public opposition in the early stages of a progressive process.

Three characteristic and diagnostic signs should alert the doctor to the possibility that his position may be compromised. Any one of them is sufficient to cause concern. The first sign is the labelling of an individual or a group in a way that implies that they are less deserving of care and comfort. Terms such as mentally defective, dangerous, violent, or terrorist are used to distance our care and concern for individuals or groups. Secondly, any restriction on the doctor's ability to publish information about his professional activities should be viewed with anxiety. In this country the Official Secrets Act severely restricts the freedom of doctors employed by the State, in particular circumstances, to publish anything which they may have seen or heard during the course of their professional duties, whether the individual doctor 'signs' it or not. Finally, any restriction of the doctor's right to make and take away independent clinical records about individual patients places the patient and doctor in a vulnerable position. The doctor may not be allowed to remove the institution's own records or the contributions which he makes to those records. Any restriction of his ability to make independent notes at his own expense puts the doctor in a position where it may be unethical to proceed.

Torture

The most serious ethical problems have been experienced in various parts of the world by doctors in relation to torture. In 1986 the BMA published the results of its world-wide enquiry into allegations of medical involvement in torture ('The Torture Report', BMA 1986). The report identified some of the conflicts for doctors in the care of their patients when basic human rights for all citizens cannot be guaranteed or even assumed. It accepted that torture is: 'The deliberate, systematic or wanton infliction of physical and mental suffering by one or more persons acting alone or on the orders of an authority, to force another person to yield information, to make confession, or for any other reason which is an outrage on personal dignity'.

In the sections which follow various situations are explored in which the doctor may face dilemmas when human rights are denied to his patients.

The BMA working party set up to consider this matter concluded that torture or brutal treatment of detained persons corrupts society and brings its administration down to the level of the violence it seeks to eradicate. The BMA considers activities by doctors which fall outside international codes of medical ethics and of international protocols to be professional misconduct. It found incontrovertible evidence ('The Torture Report' BMA 1986) of the doctors' involvement in planning and assisting in torture, not only under duress, but also voluntarily, as an exercise of the doctor's free will. A clear example of such activities includes the compulsory detention in psychiatric institutions of people whom most doctors would consider to be mentally normal and the administration of drugs which have no therapeutic purpose and which may positively harm the subject. To eradicate or limit these abuses the BMA recommends that:

1. The training of doctors should include positive guidance about the ethical framework within which doctors are expected to apply their skills and

knowledge. Such positive training should identify pressures which may be applied to distort a doctor's judgements about the moral framework within which decisions have to be taken.

2. The doctor's special duty to individuals may transcend national interest and security. The medical profession has a responsibility to support any practitioner who refuses to keep silent about abuses of human rights.

3. All deaths of citizens while detained in custody must be the subject of independent, objective and competent medico-legal autopsy even though there is no obvious reason to suspect unnatural death.

4. Doctors required to examine people detained in custody, for whatever reason, must be fully trained in detecting and evaluating signs of physical violence. Doctors should keep personal notes of the results of their examinations separate from records retained in the institution.

5. The conduct required of a doctor in respect of the examination and treatment of those detained in custody must be clear and unambiguous. The doctor must always identify himself to the prisoner and explain the reasons for the examination or treatment.

6. Doctors having knowledge of any activities covered by the Declaration of Tokyo have a positive obligation to make those activities publicly known. Each national medical association's ethical machinery must permit the prompt, efficient and objective investigation of complaints of unethical behaviour. The finding of the medical association's enquiry into unethical behaviour should be published to the whole profession of the country concerned.

7. Doctors in countries where torture does not occur have a responsibility to assist colleagues in countries where it does.

Defence of Human Rights

It can be seen from the above section that torture is much more than the physical abuse of prisoners. It is an outrage on personal dignity. It is clear from the BMA 'Torture Report' that the BMA regards any such outrage as abhorrent and the involvement of doctors, directly or indirectly, as unethical. Various attempts have been made to develop supranational principles which all States will follow. The most recent is Article 12 of the United Nations' Covenant on economic, social and cultural rights which came into force on 3 January 1976. It has been ratified, or is adhered to, by over fifty nations, and is legally binding on those nations. By seeking to provide basic human rights for all citizens the Covenant seeks to create conditions in which torture cannot occur. The most obvious area of risk is that in which the individual is deprived of his liberty. A doctor may be called to provide medical services to the prisoner or may be involved in the detention process as part of his official duties.

Duty to Protect Patients

If given the opportunity, the doctor should examine an individual on first detention even if he suspects that the detainee may subsequently be abused or tortured. The object of the examination must be to provide a base record of the individual's physical and mental health. It is less useful if the doctor is precluded from keeping his own individual notes outside the place of detention. Any involvement in the torture or abuse of a detainee is unethical and any other treatment or care after the event must be withheld until the doctor can have complete control over the treatment. The decision that recovery is complete must be that of the physician.

During the course of his duties a doctor may witness abuses (including in prisons). He may not be directly involved but may by chance have seen some incident on his way to or from his patient. The doctor will first need to assess the nature and severity of the abuse. Having decided that the matter should be pursued, the doctor will then need to decide whether to make further enquiries and possibly to register a formal protest within the organisation, or whether the matter is so serious that his protest must be registered outside the institution. It is unethical for the doctor to tolerate a situation which he knows to be wrong even if the discovery was entirely accidental.

A doctor who has become involved in a situation in which his ethical freedom is constrained should ensure that adequate arrangements exist for such ethical problems to be discussed with medical colleagues. Ideally an appeal mechanism outside the particular State-controlled system should be sought. Where this is not possible adequate professional mechanisms within the system must be provided. Without them it is unethical for a doctor to proceed. A doctor must not collude with any procedure he considers to be unethical. If he cannot act effectively to change the situation he should resign his position.

A frequent justification for the imposition of the State's wishes at the expense of the individual is the so-called doctrine of the greater good. It is argued that the individual's rights may be ignored if by so doing the freedom of many other innocent persons may be safeguarded. Such an argument has been used to justify intimate body searches of those thought to be concealing dangerous weapons and the 'interrogation' of those involved in terrorist threats. The BMA has agreed that doctors should conduct intimate body searches in order to bring such procedures within an ethical code. Doctors are invited to consult the BMA Guidelines for Intimate Body Searches (Appendix II). Doctors who participate in such procedures should take note that they are personally responsible for the decisions they take.

Similarly, no doctor may be present before, during, or after the interrogation of a prisoner. There is a notable exception to this absolute requirement, namely those who have freely volunteered to undergo training to assist them to withhold information during 'vigorous interrogation'.

The Doctor's Responsibility to the State

Many governments seek to provide care and welfare for their citizens and such provision usually includes health care. Whilst this normally produces a happier relationship between doctor and State, a note of caution may be necessary since the State's concern for its citizens may threaten individual autonomy.

Certain groups, notably police surgeons, prison medical officers and doctors serving in the Armed Forces, may experience conflict between their obligation to their employer and their responsibility to patients. Community physicians represent another group of doctors having a particular relationship with the State.

Police Surgeons

A police surgeon may not only have to examine patients on behalf of the police, but also examine and treat ill patients in custody. The doctor should be clear where his responsibilities lie. It would be improper for him to disregard the ordinary guidelines for confidentiality (ref: chapter 3) when he is treating a detained person as a patient (ref: chapter 4).

Examinations

The police surgeon should identify himself to the person to be examined and explain the purpose of the examination, and of any specimen which may be requested. The person in custody is not obliged to submit to medical examination or treatment or to provide specimens for forensic examination. In the absence of consent therefore, any treatment or attempt to obtain specimens would constitute an assault.

If the consent of the person in custody has been obtained the examination should, if possible, be witnessed by a third party. A police officer may be present but should not be within earshot. In the case of a woman in custody, a policewoman or other female should always be present (but not within earshot). If a solicitor wishes to be present during the examination the accused's consent should be obtained.

Occasions will arise when the doctor may feel it proper to disregard this advice in the interests of personal safety, but he should try to inform the patient that the confidentiality of the results of examination cannot be preserved.

It should be remembered that any consent given in custody is unlikely to be totally free from constraint.

Fitness for Custody and Observation

The information obtained on examination is confidential and only sufficient details should be given to the police to enable them to take proper care of the individual. In the cases of serious illness some information may be given, but not if the illness is the result of the patient's indiscretion, e.g. venereal disease. Information obtained as a result of observation where consent to examination has been refused may not be revealed without the consent of the accused except on the direction of a court.

Minors

Relatives may be present at the examination of a person under the age of sixteen if they request it and the minor agrees. If no relatives are available a minor may have to be placed under legal guardianship in order that consent may be obtained (ref: Chapter 4).

Unconscious Patient

Examination and essential procedures to ensure the life of a person in custody may be carried out without consent if the person is unconscious. No other procedure may be undertaken at the same time. Specimens may be taken for biochemical investigation, i.e. diagnostic purposes, but the results of tests must not be re-used for forensic purposes without the patient's subsequent consent. If the individual is under sixteen a parent or guardian can give consent to these procedures.

Prison Medical Officers

Imprisonment deprives the individual of liberty and of autonomy in varying degrees. Loss of liberty should not imply the loss of rights to medical care of a proper ethical standard.

A prisoner on remand may, through his solicitor and with the assistance of the prison medical officer, consult a doctor of his own choice. A convicted prisoner has no such freedom of choice. A prison medical officer's duty to and relationship with his patients is, however, the same as for any other doctor. He will have particular regard to the advice given on consent to treatment, research and torture.

In the course of his duties a prison medical officer will make written or verbal reports to courts, adjudication boards, prison governors, or other authorities. In the case of reports to courts, the prisoner's consent to disclosure should always be obtained. In other cases consent should be sought, but in the absence of consent the prison medical officer must be guided by his assessment of the prisoner's best interest.

Doctors in the Armed Forces

A doctor in the Armed Forces has to obey any lawful command that is given to him. Disobedience is an offence punishable by court martial. It is possible that a particular command may conflict with his ethical responsibilities. In all three services a serving doctor is responsible for his professional actions to the same extent as a civilian medical practitioner and is expected to work within the same ethical constraints as the rest of the profession. The ethical freedom of serving medical officers is guarded by the Surgeon General. He has accepted that he must ensure that no medical officer is required to treat a patient in accordance with a given policy when the doctor believes that treatment is not in that patient's best interest.

When a person joins the Armed Forces he tacitly consents to give up some of the freedoms of civilian life. One of these is the right to strict confidentiality. There are times when a medical officer is required to discuss cases with his commanding officer in the interests of the unit as a whole. If a serviceman takes his family on an accompanied posting, the health of the family may affect the serviceman and the unit. On overseas postings the family are therefore subject to the same constraints as the servicemen. The rules governing the actions of medical officers in the Armed Forces are currently under review.

The Community Physician

The community physician is employed directly or indirectly to provide independent medical advice to identified communities. Whereas in individual medical practice a person will consult the doctor who may conduct an examination, make investigations and propose a course of treatment, the community physician has an analogous relationship to the group of people for whom he has accepted professional responsibility. He may examine the community, undertake investigations and recommend a course of action to alleviate a problem which has been identified. Yet the community articulates its wishes largely through its leaders, who for economic, political or other reasons may wish to limit the community physician's role or oppose his recommended solution. The community physician must inevitably sacrifice some of his professional autonomy by the nature of his employment. The specialty remains divided between those who demand an advisory role as independent consult- ants, without responsibility for implementing the recommended solution, and those who believe that involvement in its implementation is essential despite the inevitable constraints which involvement will bring.

To maintain an ethical stance, community physicians must retain a right to make a direct appeal to the community itself and not just to its leaders. If the community is the 'patient', no-one has the right to withhold proposed treatment without the community being aware of this fact. Secondly, the community physician always needs to be able to communicate with the community's leaders and not merely their officers and managers. No inter- ference in this line of communication is acceptable. There has been worrying evidence in recent years that both these principles are being eroded.

Community physicians are usually employed by health authorities but many are also required to give professional advice to other public authorities. In some cases the community physician may be given statutory powers by a local authority to discharge certain functions under the Public Health Act (Control of Diseases) 1984. The separation of his professional responsibility from his employment status should provide a valuable safeguard for this ethical duty to speak out on health issues affecting the community for which he is responsible. In practice these quite separate roles are confused by employing authorities, so that the community physician may find his ability to provide independent medical advice seriously compromised. His ethical duty to the local community is not diminished by confusion about the nature of his role.

The community physician is required to interpret information, sometimes clinical information, which is already held by managers and authority members. The ethical responsibility is to ensure that wrong deductions are not made from such information.

Similarly the community physician has a duty of confidentiality. Part of his professional role may involve information about individual patients. While he may interpret and act upon such information, it remains subject to the ethical requirement of confidentiality. Indeed, if the analogy between the patient and the community is to be properly understood, it is clear that the community physician may also receive management information because of his privileged position which he has an ethical responsibility to keep confidential. This may occasionally present him with the embarrassing situation in which he has a duty to disclose his proposed solution, whilst keeping confidential the information on which it was based. In resolving such conflicts community physicians should seek to keep themselves in close touch with the general ethical conduct of the profession as a whole.

Doctors in the Health Care System

In this country the State has largely undertaken to meet the cost of health care, but this introduces a significant new factor into the relationship between doctor and patient. The State is entitled to decide how much of the health care it is prepared to provide or pay for, to decide whether it is receiving value for its money and to assess the effectiveness of the care which the patient receives.

The doctor working within such a health care system needs to be aware of cost effectiveness as well as clinical effectiveness in the care provided for the patient, including consideration of suitable treatment options. The doctor is under some obligation to provide information which will assist others to estimate the costs of care provided.

The doctor has a clear ethical obligation to honour all the contractual responsibilities placed on him by the health care system in which he has agreed to participate. This may include the level of service which he has undertaken to give, or his duty as an employee to work the number of hours which he has contracted to undertake.

At times there may be conflicts between the patient's needs and the needs or priorities of the health care system. The doctor must remember that at all times the patient's welfare and best interests must remain paramount in his thinking. Those doctors working as community physicians, or undertaking administrative or supervisory duties within management, may have a different ethical responsibility in relation to the same patient.

These issues are discussed at greater length on pages 71–73.

Doctors in Management Posts

In the last two years, several doctors have been appointed to management posts either full-time or part-time. This inevitably creates a conflict of roles a useful example of which is the receipt of information. A doctor in management may receive information solely because he is a doctor and that information may be useful to him in making a management decision. Nevertheless, the information itself remains privileged to him as a doctor and he has an ethical responsibility to preserve its confidentiality. Such dilemmas occur in many other management situations and it is important for the doctor to ensure that his management position never places him in a position where he can no longer exercise his primary responsibility to individual patients in his charge.

There is a great need for doctors to be trained in management techniques and particularly in the ethical conflicts which occur in management. It cannot be assumed that management is always pursued with the same regard for integrity, honesty and loyalty on which the doctor's professional status depends. Doctors entering management need to understand the pressures which are likely to be placed on them performing their new duties.

A system of individual performance review has been introduced for all those occupying managerial positions in the NHS. This system is increasingly being associated with financial rewards and penalties and it can only accentuate the dilemmas of medical managers.

6 Doctors Practising in Special Communities

There are other special circumstances where doctors may be working in relation to defined population groups. Here difficulties may arise in the responsibility to the employer or to a particular community, and the care of the individual patient.

In all these situations the other members of the community should understand the doctor's role. By the very nature of their participation in that community, these members accept modification of the normal rules of confidentiality. This does not mean that the doctor has no requirement of confidentiality but it does mean that he can be forced by the rules of the job, or his perception of what is necessary for the good of the community as a whole, to reveal information which would otherwise be kept confidential, and this should be included in the contract of employment.

Ships' Surgeons and Expedition Doctors

Ships' surgeons, medical officers in the Merchant Navy and doctors who are members of an expedition work in an environment that is similar to that of Armed Forces doctors. They all work in a situation where the community may be put at risk if the community as a whole or at least the leader or Captain is unaware that a member of the crew, the team or a passenger is either a risk to the community through an illness or is incapable of carrying out some vital task because of illness. The doctor must decide in such circumstances that unless the damage to his patient will be out of proportion to the risk of giving the information then his duty to the community as a whole will oblige him to divulge what he believes is necessary.

Occupational Health Physicians

Occupational Medicine

Occupational medicine is that specialty which deals with the effects of work on health and health on work. The occupational physician must act as an impartial professional adviser, concerned with safeguarding the health of all those employed in the organisation by whom he is appointed. Although he is normally appointed and paid by the management his duties concern the health

45

and welfare of all the workforce both individually and collectively. The reader is referred to the Advisory Conciliation and Arbitration Service (ACAS) code of practice 'Disciplinary Practice and Procedures in Employment', and the Royal College of Physicians Faculty of Occupational Medicine's 'Guidance on Ethics for Occupational Physicians, Dec 1986'.

Intra-professional relations

In most circumstances he is dealing with the patients of other doctors, as are most hospital medical staff. Normally, with the individual's agreement, the patient's own general practitioner should be informed of relevant clinical information which comes to the attention of the occupational physician.

When the occupational physician is seeking further clinical details from the general practitioner or from hospital medical staff he should obtain the patient's written agreement and consent.

The occupational physician should, except in an emergency, treat patients only in co-operation with the patient's general practitioner. This applies also to the use of special facilities or other staff (e.g. occupational health nurses, physiotherapists) whom he may have in his department.

In an emergency the occupational physician may refer a patient to a hospital or a consultant. He should inform the patient's general practitioner of any such action taken.

Occupational physicians should not influence any employee in his choice of general practitioner. If he believes that the employee should consult his general practitioner he should urge him to do so.

Visits by other doctors or nurses (including consultants in occupational medicine, Employment Medical or Nursing Advisers, general practitioners and other specialists) to industrial, commercial or other workplaces should be subject to proper professional courtesy. The visiting doctor or nurse should make every effort to identify the occupational physician to the company (whether part-time or full-time) and inform him in advance of his intention to visit the factory or workplace, preferably at a time when the occupational physician can be present.

Sickness Absence

The occupational physician does not usually have to confirm or refute that absence from work is due to sickness or injury. If the occupational physician wishes to assess the fitness for work of an employee who is still absent for health reasons, he should consult the general practitioner with the written consent of the patient.

On an employee's return to work the occupational physician is responsible for advice to management on the worker's fitness for the job and may be asked to advise on any work or time restrictions to be arranged whether temporary or permanent. He should seek the patient's consent before advising management of important job changes. He should inform the patient of the advice he is to give to management.

In cases where an employee's sickness absence record is prolonged or excessive the occupational physician may be asked to advise both employee and employer on future employability. While the employer has no right to clinical details of sickness or injury, the doctor he employs can reasonably be expected to advise the employer on the implications of those clinical facts and opinions in terms of:

(a) the likely date of return to work – if any;

(b) the likely degree of disability of the patient at the time of return to work;

(c) the likely duration of that disability;

(d) the relevance of any underlying condition to the absence record;

(e) the likelihood of regular and efficient service in the future.

The decision to take action against an employee who has had excessive absence from work is the prerogative of management. However, the occupational physician should remember that he may have to give evidence to an industrial tribunal in such cases (see medical records below).

In cases of retirement on medical grounds the occupational physician should inform the patient's general practitioner of the advice he has given whether to the employer or to the pensions department where this is relevant.

Medical Records

The responsibility for confidentiality of clinical records is that of the occupational physician and the occupational health nurse with whom they are shared. The fact that the doctor is employed by an organisation does not mean that the employer or the employee or his representative has any right to see the results of examinations or notes written by the doctor or nurse.

If an employer requires a medical opinion on a member of his staff, the employee should be aware of the reason for that management referral, and of the need for a subsequent medical report to management.

The occupational physician should inform the employee about the substance of any subsequent report to management.

Naturally, clinical records may also need to be seen by clerical support staff and secretaries. The occupational physician must ensure that those people are placed under contractual obligation to preserve the confidentiality of the records.

In questions of litigation, clinical records of patients or abstracts or summaries from them should not be released without the patient's written consent (see

47

Chapter 4). Confidential medical records may be released by a valid order of a properly constituted Court, or by an industrial tribunal. In the event of the doctor refusing he risks being held in contempt of Court (see Chapter 3 – Confidentiality).

Arrangement must be made for proper transfer of medical records to another physician or occupational health nurse when the occupational physician leaves for any reason, or retires or dies. If the records cannot be properly safeguarded they should be destroyed.

In the case of occupational injury or disease the occupational physician may provide the legal advisers of both employer and employee (with the latter's written consent) with factual information about dates and times of attendances at medical departments and about first aid and other treatment.

Medical Examinations

The occupational physician and/or occupational health nurse frequently perform routine examinations to determine the fitness of individuals for a particular job. Some of these examinations are required by statute (e.g. heavy goods vehicle, public service vehicle drivers, airline pilots), some are required by the industries (e.g. food handlers) and some by the company (e.g. pre-employment). It could be inferred from the applicant's attendance that he agrees both to the examination and to the disclosure of the result. Nevertheless the doctor and nurse should in these circumstances make clear to the individual their roles in performing these examinations and that the results (without clinical details) will be given to the employer.

Periodic medical examinations which may include special investigations such as radiographic or biochemical tests are required for workers exposed to certain hazards. Individual clinical findings are confidential though their significance may be conveyed to a third party. Thus while an individual result may not be published it may be proper to disclose (as may be required by statute) that a work group shows a significant degree of exposure to a potentially toxic hazard.

Commercial Secrecy

Employers and manufacturers are required to disclose information about a process or product which may constitute a risk to health at the place of work (Health and Safety at Work, etc Act 1974 sections 6 and 2(2c)). In the course of his work an occupational physician may come into possession of confidential information about a commercial process or product. If he can establish that the process may be harmful to health, and if he has failed to persuade the employer to release such information, he should consult in confidence his professional colleagues. His responsibility for the health of workers both in the factory and elsewhere exposed to hazard should take precedence over the management's refusal to disclose but he must always tell management what steps he proposes to take.

A possible solution will be to seek the advice of the Employment Medical Advisory Service but it should be understood that the latter may be under a legal obligation to disclose the circumstances to the Health and Safety Executive. In the last resort the occupational physician may have to warn the workers himself and face the consequences.

7 The European States and the European Community (EC)

The directives relating to the free movement of doctors in the EC impose on a doctor who migrates the duty to conform to the ethical code of the host country. Some aspects of medical ethics are not identical in the countries of the EC, and the UK style of practice is by no means universal. The ethical duties of doctors are frequently incorporated as codes within national legislation. In European law the preambles set out clearly the objectives of the legislation.

Other EC countries may regulate areas of medical practice which are not normally the concern of the General Medical Council in the UK, such as the conditions of contract between a doctor and a hospital or the conditions under which doctors may form a group. The notable exception to the situation in the old six members of the original European Community is that of the Netherlands, where no detailed ethical code appears in national legislation. The Law only places on the doctor the duty to conduct himself so as to retain the confidence of his patients, to ensure his professional competence and to observe professional secrecy except where the law provides for disclosure.

Recently the Conference Internationale des Ordres et des Organismes d'Attributions Similaires, a body comprising representatives of the regulatory bodies of the member states of the European Community has drawn up a European ethical guide, entitled 'Principles of Medical Ethics in Europe'.

In the UK this code has now been considered by the GMC. It is not an ethical code but a set of guiding principles which may be of help to doctors considering difficult ethical problems. Other member states are also considering what status to give the 'code'.

The rigid application of the principles of confidentiality or secrecy is a marked feature of all ethical systems in the six countries of the original EC, whereas a UK doctor may refuse to disclose information about his patients at his peril. Only at the discretion of the Court may a UK doctor withhold information about his patients. The Courts may order him to disclose information, and should he refuse he is at risk of being held in contempt of Court. In the original EC countries (the old six), however, medical secrecy is much more firmly protected by the Law.

UK doctors are regarded by their European colleagues as having gone a long way towards abandoning the 'absolute secrecy' which they defend. Indeed, to breach confidentiality is a criminal offence in some countries; this shows the importance attached to it. There exist in all countries certain derogations from this principle of absolute secrecy but codes which superficially appear similar may have significant differences. For example, the Belgian code does not permit the doctor to be released from his duty to safeguard secrecy even when the patient has expressly given his permission. Other principles upon which the European codes are based include:

In relation to the general principles underlying medical practice:

(a) Respect for life.

(b) Equality of patients regardless of religion, race or reputation.

(c) The obligation to provide emergency care and to ensure the continuity of care.

(d) Regard for the independence of the profession.

(e) Respect for the dignity of the profession which must not be undermined.

(f) The prohibition of all commercial practices and all activity incompatible with the dignity of the profession.

(g) Professional secrecy.

In relation to social security systems:

(a) Free choice of doctor by the patient.

(b) Freedom of the doctor to prescribe.

(c) Direct negotiations between doctor and patient concerning fees.

(d) Direct payment of fees by the patient to the doctor.

The Standing Committee of Doctors in the EC (CP), founded in 1959, which represents the medical profession within the European Community, has among its committees one dealing with ethics and one dealing with social security. Among the charters prepared and endorsed by the CP is that of Nuremburg (1980) dealing with the practice of medicine in the Community, which details the fundamental rights of patients and doctors (reproduced in the chapter on Ethical Codes and Statements), and declarations on health care costs, the right to strike and 'in vitro' fertilisation.

The European Union of General Practitioners (UEMO) has been particularly concerned with the safeguarding of confidentiality, especially in relation to the use of data banks, and has drawn up a list of principles to be observed when medical information is stored in this way (reproduced in the chapter on Ethical Codes and Statements).

8 Professional Behaviour

Doctors are expected to behave with honour and probity towards patients, other doctors and the rest of society. The doctor's primary responsibility is to patients and their best interests must be put above all other considerations. When a doctor is registered and begins to practise medicine he accepts these expectations and knows that by behaving in accordance with them he will earn society's respect and be given the trust which will admit him into situations not open to others. Without such respect and trust the doctor/patient relationship is of little value. A high standard of professional behaviour is therefore essential. Unprofessional behaviour by any medical practitioner puts at risk the standing of all medical practitioners.

Medical students and doctors in training are learning and it is the responsibility of all doctors to teach what they know to them. Much training is done by letting them carry out delegated tasks under supervision. The principles that apply to such delegation are the same as those applying to all forms of delegation of medical tasks, including deputising arrangements. It is unethical to delegate work to another health professional unless he is suitably qualified and experienced to undertake that work (for the General Medical Council's view, see 'Professional Conduct and Discipline: Fitness to Practise', paragraphs 40 et seq). The teaching doctor or trainer is responsible for acquainting himself with the competence of his student or trainee and for allowing him to deputise only within his competence.

General practitioners who use a deputising service are effectively unable to exercise any direct choice of deputy and must rely on the management of the service to choose staff of appropriate competence. They have a duty, however, to inform the management of untoward incidents so that action can be taken to avoid any recurrence. Some deputising services are controlled solely by doctors, but most are controlled jointly by a commercial organisation and the profession.

It has been customary in the past and obligatory since 1978 for there to be a professional advisory committee connected with each deputising service to ensure that clinical and organisational standards are maintained. This should help principals in the NHS using such services to feel satisfied that the deputies will be of an adequate standard.

Medical care cannot be limited to conventional working hours, but a doctor cannot be on duty continuously without detriment to the quality of his work and his health. Deputising or delegating arrangements must not jeopardise the patient's welfare and for these arrangements to be ethically acceptable two conditions must be satisfied. First, the doctor who has been chosen and accepted by the patient should ensure as far as practicable that the deputy is experienced, competent, conscientious and in other respects suitable to perform the delegated responsibilities of the usual doctor. Secondly, there must be adequate communications and record systems to permit proper treatment both during and after the deputising period. These principles apply to delegation to locums, cross-cover between specialties and to delegation to junior staff within the same specialty. They apply to doctors working in general practice and to trainees in community medicine.

A fully registered practitioner is responsible not only to those who employ or delegate responsibility to him, but also to each patient. Provisionally registered practitioners carry the same responsibility within the hospital where they are employed. Such doctors in training have a responsibility to take account of the advice of their consultants or general practice trainer. If a doctor believes that the general advice he has been given is not applicable to a particular situation, or not in the best interests of an individual patient, he should seek further specific advice. If necessary he should ask the consultant or general practitioner to take back their delegated authority and take over the management of the patient's illness personally. The primary responsibility of a junior doctor in a training post is to the patient; he should decline to do anything that he believes is not in the patient's best interests.

Doctors must act in the best interests of their patients. As professionals, they must be reliable and honest. Because of this doctors are relied upon to sign documents and certificates. A doctor should be aware that his signature on a document or a certificate validates the information or opinion contained in it. He must exercise care in issuing certificates and similar documents and should not include in them statements that he has not taken appropriate steps to verify. No doctor should sign a document without fully checking the contents of that document. If a doctor in civilian practice or serving with the Armed Forces feels unable to sign a certificate indicating fitness for a prospective event, it is proper for him to record whether, at the time of examination, the subject was healthy or not.

For some years it has been thought that signing routine forms such as those produced by a haematological counter means only that the doctor is satisfied that the equipment is operating within satisfactory quality control limits. His signature does not validate the information on an individual form, for he lacks knowledge of the particular specimen. It should be noted however that it is likely that the Courts would treat the doctor's signature as affirming the veracity of the information which he has personally ascertained. However, he remains responsible for any opinion or comment that he expresses upon the results. Where a computer makes comments on a form the doctor is signing he should satisfy himself that the computed comment is consistent with the data upon which that comment is based. He is then taking responsibility for that comment as if he had made it himself.

Because the doctor bears a primary responsibility to the patient he must not be seen to be acting in collusion with other doctors to further his own interests at the expense of patients. In particular the secret division by two or more doctors of fees on a basis of commission, or some other defined method of fee splitting is a practice that has brought the profession into disrepute on a number of occasions. Any undisclosed division of professional fees, except in a medical partnership publicly known to exist, is unethical.

Doctors should always attempt to treat other doctors as colleagues and not interfere with their colleagues' relationships with their patients or each other. However, from time to time doctors working together in a practice or in the same locality find themselves in disagreement, or one may feel that another has not been behaving professionally. It is important that disputes be resolved quickly and amicably within the profession itself. If animosities are allowed to fester they not only embitter local practice but also damage the profession's reputation. If a doctor has information about a colleague which may raise a question of serious professional misconduct he has an ethical duty to seek the advice of the GMC. Most such disagreements do not concern questions of professional misconduct but are based upon the traditions of the profession. Members of the BMA may obtain advice from their local divisions or from the Central Ethical Committee as to how these disagreements should be settled. If this advice fails to resolve the situation, there are detailed uniform rules of procedure for the investigation of complaints. The full procedure can be obtained from the BMA but is outlined below.

The preliminary stage requires the complainant to write to the respondent (stating the complaint in terms specific enough to enable the respondent to reply) saying that he is considering beginning a complaint through the BMA's ethical machinery, and inviting his reply. A copy of the letter of complaint, and any reply must be submitted to the Honorary Secretary of the appropriate Division of the Association. The Honorary Secretary then sends the correspondence to the Head Office and obtains instructions on the steps to be taken to deal with the matter. If Head Office so instructs, the Honorary Secretary refers it to the Division's Ethical Committee. This Committee should be established in each Division at its AGM.

The Divisional Ethical Committee will consider the matter having heard from both parties to the dispute and will attempt to resolve the situation. If this is unsuccessful then the matter will be referred to the Central Ethical Committee which will convey its opinion back to the Division. It is up to the Division to consider the opinions of the local or Central Ethical Committee. Having done so it will post to the parties concerned any resolutions that have been passed as a result of their deliberations.

Sick Doctors

Attention should be drawn to the fact that there is now a voluntary national counselling scheme for doctors in whose case, it appears to colleagues, a question arises as to their fitness to practise, on health grounds.

The General Medical Council has a statutory responsibility to take appropriate action in respect of registered practitioners in whose case information is provided in the appropriate form raising such a question.

The final relationship between doctors to be considered is the special situation which arises when a doctor is being seen as a patient. When a doctor consults another doctor as a patient it is a mark of respect for the doctor consulted since the choice of the consulting doctor is a much more informed choice than that of any other patient. There is a long-standing tradition that in private practice a doctor should not charge another doctor for treatment or advice to that doctor or his immediate dependant relatives. Every effort should be made to maintain the traditional practice of the medical profession whereby attendance by one doctor upon another or upon his dependants is without direct charge. There has been a recent trend away from this tradition. This trend is to be deplored and was overwhelmingly rejected at the 1986 ARM of the BMA when a motion was put forward to end it. It is perfectly acceptable to receive a gift from a colleague you have treated but ethically unacceptable to send a bill.

9 The Doctor and the Media

Increasing public interest in health matters has brought doctors more and more into contact with the news media. It is therefore essential that doctors should be aware of the ethics of dealing with the media.

Those doctors able to comment authoritatively on medical subjects should be prepared to do so in order that the public may be informed. Those doctors able to help the public with information should regard talking to the media as an extension of their medical practice. They must, however, ensure that they observe the basic ethical guidance in relation to advertising.

A doctor has the responsibility to ensure that when a subject under discussion is controversial within the medical profession, the producer or editor is made aware of that fact.

It is unacceptable for a doctor publicly to discuss his own ability in a particular field in such a way as to imply that his methods are superior to those of other doctors.

If a doctor receives an individual medical enquiry following a report in the media he may acknowledge the enquiry, but should refer the patient to his usual medical practitioner.

Identification of the Doctor

It is acceptable for the doctor's identity to be revealed in the following circumstances:

– when it does not add to his professional stature;

– when it is in the public interest, such as an announcement by a community physician about an outbreak of a communicable disease;

– when he is speaking on behalf of an identifiable section of the profession;

– when using media primarily aimed at doctors.

A doctor may use his own name in connection with subjects other than medicine.

When discussing a medical subject in the lay press, or on radio or television, he may be named only if he confines himself to general terms, avoiding discussion of identifiable individual cases.

Doctors making statements on behalf of known organisations may be named when this is in the public interest. However, a doctor must not exploit the media to promote any organisation in which he has a financial interest.

A doctor contributing his professional or clinical views in the media should make clear any economic interest he may have in the subject.

10 Gifts and Hospitality

The public has a right to be concerned if they feel that professional advice offered to them may have been influenced by financial or other benefits offered to professionals by commercial organisations whose products or services are being recommended by those professionals. The medical profession has an obligation to assure the public that treatment offered is appropriate and is justified by its intrinsic merit, uninfluenced by commercial or financial interests. This is especially important in relation to pharmaceutical products.

The balance is very delicate and with increasing public concern there has been greater demand for definition of strict guidelines both for the medical profession, as to what is acceptable, and for the pharmaceutical industry, concerning what it may offer to the medical profession. The area of clinical drug trials is particularly delicate in this respect (see Chapter 14 – Research). Joint advice has been issued by the BMA and others on subjects such as 'Clinical Trials in General Practice' and 'Post Marketing Surveillance' (available from the General Medical Services Committee of the BMA).

On at least two occasions the European Community Authorities have interested themselves in this subject, being critical mainly of the promotion of pharmaceutical products. Nevertheless they also recognise the substantial role played by the pharmaceutical industry in assisting research and assisting Continuing Medical Education.

The DHSS has issued a Health Note (HN(62)21) about gifts and hospitality, drawing the attention of hospital staff to the Prevention of Corruption Acts 1906 and 1916. Independent contractors, e.g. general practitioners, are not under any contractual duty to comply with the instructions of this note as they are not employees. However, they, like all other citizens, are subject to the provisions of the Prevention of Corruption Act 1906 and 1916 and they would therefore be wise to consider the underlying principles, as in the Health Note.

As prescribers of pharmaceutical products, they also have an ethical responsibility to satisfy themselves that their prescribing is responsible.

These basic principles concerning inducements apply equally to doctors who are working in private general or psychiatric hospitals.

If the doctor can honestly state that regardless of any promotional activity, his judgement when prescribing adheres to the criteria mentioned above then he is acting ethically. In relation to Research and Evaluation the independent contractor will of course have to satisfy himself that the appropriate information about the financing of any research trial is included in the protocol documentation submitted to the local ethical committee.

The principle on which this chapter is based is whether or not those employed by the State are in fact influenced by promotional (as opposed to educational) material or incentives. They must be seen to be above influence. As far as the 'independent health professional', e.g. the general practitioner, is concerned, the situation is substantially different, but the basic principle remains unaltered. As a profession, doctors must be seen to be uninfluenced by any non-scientific promotion directed towards them by the pharmaceutical industry.

The degree to which individual doctors may be influenced by promotion of pharmaceutical products varies considerably. Some doctors may accept relatively uncritically the presentations by the pharmaceutical industry; others critically analyse the presentations and published literature. Those who have conducted trials on drugs may be expected to have analysed the advantage and risk factors carefully regardless of the presentation of the product by the industry.

There does not appear to have been extensive analysis of the degree to which doctors may be subliminally influenced by promotional methods used by the industry.

It must be recognized that the substantial support of the pharmaceutical industry in promoting Continuing Medical Education has been of benefit not only to the industry but also to the profession and patients.

Whether a doctor prescribes a new product or not must clearly depend on his scientific and clinical integrity when considering the information provided by the company.

Promotional activities to individuals, however, may raise serious ethical problems. The pharmaceutical industry recognises this and the Association of British Pharmaceutical Industry have a strict Code of Practice (reproduced in the Data Sheet Compendium) which refers specifically to the acceptable practice concerning gifts and hospitality. The Royal College of Physicians has also examined this question in their publication 'Relationships between the profession and the pharmaceutical industry'. Doctors would be well advised to consider the degree to which they may compromise themselves when an offer is of such a nature as to put at risk their ability to defend themselves against the accusation of being unreasonably influenced. The GMC offers the following advice from its booklet 'Professional Conduct and Discipline: Fitness to Practice April 1987':

'It may be improper for an individual doctor to accept from a pharmaceutical firm monetary gifts or loans of expensive items of equipment for his personal use. No exception can, however, be taken to grants of money or equipment by firms to institutions such as hospitals, health care centres and university departments, when they are donated specifically for purposes of research.

It may be improper for individual doctors or groups of doctors to accept lavish hospitality or travel facilities under the terms of sponsorship of medical postgraduate meetings or conferences. However, no exception is likely to be taken to acceptance by an individual doctor of a grant which enables him to travel to an international conference or to acceptance, by a group of doctors who attend a sponsored postgraduate meeting or conference, of hospitality at an appropriate level, which the recipients might normally adopt when paying for themselves'.

11 Establishing a Practice

General Practice

A doctor may set up in NHS general practice by appointment to a partnership, or to a single-handed practice vacancy. Under NHS regulations the sale of goodwill is illegal, but private practitioners may purchase the goodwill of an existing practice. In either case, a doctor may establish a new practice in certain circumstances.

A general practitioner notifying patients of a change of address, or surgery hours, may send a sealed letter to patients of the practice. A suitable notice may be displayed on his premises. It is not normal practice to use the media except to place a brief notice in the local press stating the change of address, and only then if all the practitioners in the area agree. Information in any such announcement should be limited to the practitioner's name, medical qualifications, and brief details of address, hours and telephone numbers.

Specialist Practice

A doctor establishing any form of specialist practice, changing his area of practice or altering his practice arrangements must not make a public announcement. He may notify those practitioners whom he might normally expect to be interested by sending a sealed letter listing his specialty, name, address and telephone number.

Further notices may be sent out only if these arrangements are changed.

Premises: General Practice

Although the sharing of premises with members of allied professions (including those supplementary to medicine) has been discouraged in the past, advances, changes in practice and altered expectations of patients have contributed to a closer integration of services in the interests of patients.

Reference has been made elsewhere to the importance of the patient's autonomy and freedom of choice. This must be reflected in the choice practitioners make in the location and arrangement of their premises. Some may be located in large buildings. In these circumstances the sharing of facilities with organisations providing extensive commercial public use is discouraged, and practices should ensure that access to the practice team can be made via a separate entrance.

While it is important that patients should know the locations of general practitioners' premises, it is essential that door plates, notices and signposts should inform rather than advertise. The following criteria must be observed:

– a sign or plate should be unostentatious in size and form;

– details should be restricted to the doctor's name, qualifications, and surgery hours.

– it is acceptable to use languages commonly spoken in the area;

– signs should be limited to the minimum number required;

– notices should not seek to emphasise the existence of one practice at the expense of another.

In selecting the name for a health centre or medical centre, or the collective title for a partnership or association of doctors, the guidance of the GMC should be borne in mind that it is undesirable that any name chosen should carry an implication that the premises have received recognition denied to other practices locally. This is important for doctors establishing practice in premises owned by a health authority.

Premises: Specialist Practice

The sharing of premises between doctors, whether of similar or different specialties, is acceptable. However, caution is required in any arrangements that could be misinterpreted. The general practitioner should remember that patients' freedom of choice should not be compromised by any suggestion of direction, whether implicit or explicit. In particular, general practitioners should not normally share premises with those in specialist practice.

Advertising and Publicity

It is a long-held ethical principle that the medical profession should refrain from self-promotion. This is not only incompatible with the criteria governing intra-professional relationships, but could be a source of danger to the public.

Similarly, canvassing for the purpose of obtaining patients is unethical.

Patients are entitled to be given accurate information about the medical services available to them. There is a great difference between providing factual details which assist patient choice, and self-promotion. Any entry of a doctor's name in a telephone directory should appear in ordinary small type, never in a special type-face. Doctors' names may also appear in the yellow pages and in any other local registers, providing that these are open to all practitioners in the area concerned, and that no fee is required for the entry.

Information about NHS general practitioners is available from the Medical Lists published by Family Practitioner Committees. Details are listed in a nationally agreed and uniform format.

In addition, there is a welcome trend within general practice to produce 'in-house' practice leaflets. It is good practice for partnerships and practices to provide accurate, non-promotional and factual information about their services. Such literature should not draw attention to the achievements, educational or otherwise, of the doctors or the practice as a whole.

Leaflets may be made available to prospective patients. They may contain the following information:

– the practice address, telephone number and out-of-hours contact;

– the names of all the doctors in the practice;

– appointment and consulting arrangements;

– arrangements for home visit requests;

– emergency arrangements;

– the availability of special clinics;

– the practice area;

– information about the presence of students or trainees, with a reminder about the freedom of choice concerning privacy.

Commercial

[See also General Medical Council Booklet, 'Professional Conduct and Discipline: Fitness to Practise', Paragraphs 105–106 1987]

A doctor must not involve himself with commerce in such a way that it influences, or may appear to influence, his attitude towards the care of his patients.

Advertising in the lay press of nursing homes and other institutions where medical treatment is not undertaken is a well established and acceptable custom. However, as organisations providing specialist medical care should not, as a rule, accept self-referred patients, it is not necessary for private hospitals and other lay-owned organisations providing such services to advertise to the public.

A doctor involved with any organisation which advertises medical services to the public should satisfy himself that the advertising is accurate and truthful. It is undesirable for practitioners to be associated with organisations that undertake strident campaigns, or which encourage self-referral.

If a doctor has a financial interest involving his possible gain in any institution to which he refers a patient, he should disclose this fact to the patient.

If a doctor is asked to write any commentary on a commercial product to any manufacturer, especially one connected with medicine, he must ensure that his name is not used for commercial purposes.

12 Intra-professional Relationships

This chapter aims to put into context the doctor's relationships with other professionals. In an era of increasing specialisation in relation to the overall care of the patient the doctor works with other professionals whether qualified health professionals or not. These trained individuals have a function in relation to the care of the patient and the health care team but are not always bound by a professional code of ethics.

In the health care team the doctor is responsible for the medical treatment and management of the patient. As a result of this responsibility he is the key member of the team and usually heads it. Nevertheless he must recognise that other team members have skills which they may exercise without reference to the doctor. In exercising these skills they are professionally responsible for their actions.

Nurses and midwives belong to professions and have their own statutory status, standards and expertise. In cases of medical treatment nurses are obliged to follow a doctor's instructions, except where they have reason to believe that harm will be caused to the patient by so doing. In such cases nurses are obliged to communicate this to the doctor in charge of the case.

There are cases when a nurse may be more aware of the needs of a patient than a doctor; the relationship between nurses and doctors should be based on a respect for each other's area of expertise and the professional development of the nurse within the framework of the doctor's ultimate responsibility. However, a doctor would be wise to bear in mind his professional responsibilities and that it is unethical for a doctor to delegate work unless he is satisfied of the person's competence. Equally if a nurse or any other qualified health professional assumes, without delegation, professional responsibility for an action for which they have not been trained, the doctor is not ethically responsible for that action. It is nevertheless important for communication to be maintained.

A trained and registered midwife has a legal right to deliver total care on her own responsibility to a woman and her baby during the antenatal, intranatal, postnatal and neonatal periods provided that complications are neither present nor arise. Most practising midwives work within the maternity services team in the hospitals, general practitioner units and in the community.

A midwife is required to call in a registered medical practitioner in accordance with the Nurses, Midwives and Health Visitors rules (NM and HV) 1983 if complications are present or arise at any time. In such cases she is required to carry out the instructions of the doctor in attendance.

The NM and HV Rules 1983 require a midwife to ensure that before undertaking treatment outside her province or for which she has not previously been trained, she receives the necessary training and considers herself to be competent. Therefore if a doctor wishes to delegate responsibilities to a midwife which are outside her normal sphere of practice she will expect to receive the necessary instruction.

Under the Professions Supplementary to Medicine Act 1960, each of the professions has a Board and a disciplinary committee. The professions are: chiropodists, dietitians, medical laboratory scientific officers (MLSOs) (formerly laboratory technicians who do not treat patients), occupational therapists, orthoptists, physiotherapists, radiographers and remedial gymnasts. In these cases the doctor has overall responsibility for such treatment generally but not for the fine details which a reasonable doctor would not be expected to check or supervise.

The Disciplinary Statement of each Board underlines the maintenance of high standards of professional conduct. A doctor should make sure that the people to whom he refers patients are professionally registered, and that he refers patients properly to them and retains final authority for the continuation or otherwise of the therapy.

Retail pharmacists have always given informal advice to patients and are increasingly being encouraged to take an active role. Conversely, in rural dispensing practices general practitioners undertake most of the work usually done by a pharmacist. It would be unethical for a doctor to ask a pharmacist to undertake work beyond his competence, but he should recognise the pharmacist's special knowledge of drugs and of their side effects and interactions.

Collusion between doctors and others for financial gain is reprehensible. A particular example of this is collusion between doctors and pharmacists. A doctor should not arrange a commission from a pharmacist, nor should he hold a financial interest in any pharmacy in the area of his practice. Professional cards should not be handed to pharmacists for distribution. It is undesirable that messages for a doctor be received or left at pharmacies.

Co-operation between doctors and other health professionals must be based on adequate knowledge, but shared information must be treated as confidential.

Social workers and clinical psychologists are the other two professions most often present at multi-disciplinary team work. Neither profession has a professional code which is binding upon all the members. However, certain professional organisations have developed codes of conduct binding upon their own members. Until such codes are binding on all members of the professions, this affects the doctor's ability to share information and to ensure confidentiality.

The patient can benefit from collaboration between the doctor and hospital chaplains and other spiritual advisers. Patients' spiritual needs vary greatly and their wishes must be paramount. Spiritual advisers who work in hospitals gain special experience in dealing with health professionals. The patient's own spiritual adviser has special knowledge of his family and social background from which the doctor may derive special insights, especially for long-stay patients, cases of terminal illness, and of bereavement, which the doctor could usefully employ in the patient's overall clinical care.

13 Resource Allocation and Reduction of Services to Patients

The doctor/patient relationship is based on an implicit understanding by the patient that the doctor will be acting in his best interests. Patients believe that the necessary equipment and facilities will be provided to ensure a high standard of medical care irrespective of whether this care is received under the NHS, by insurance or by direct payment. This belief is not always borne out in fact.

Doctors have, in different times and places, had to contend with inadequate resources. Never is this more obvious than in wartime. Constraints placed on doctors working on a battlefield have led them to adopt the pragmatic approach of triage. This system distinguishes between those whose injuries might benefit from receiving such attention as is available, those whose injuries are relatively trivial and those who are likely to die irrespective of any treatment given. The profession and public alike tend to assume that in times of peace such problems will not arise. A possible modern application of the principles of triage is explored in the BMA discussion document 'Nuclear Attack: Ethics and Casualty Selection'.

In recent years problems of resource allocation within the National Health Service have increasingly cast doubt on this assumption. The resources allocated by Parliament to the social security system are related to the importance attached by the party in power to the NHS and social security benefits and to the overall amount of money available for the public sector. Doctors should draw the government's attention to advances in medicine, their worth and their relevance to the NHS. The government then decides on the allocation of resources. Such allocations do not always reflect the health professions' assessment of the needs of the NHS. This raises a dilemma which seems likely to persist in that there are two sets of responsibilities which can be incompatible. The profession has an ethical responsibility to provide the best possible treatment, while the State will apportion the resources for the health services from the total budget available to it on criteria other than the needs of patients. This is a growing problem. Advances in science, medicine and technology have tended to increase public expectation of better health. As more disease can be arrested or cured and developments are well publicised, patients tend to believe that their own illnesses will be cured.

The demand on the NHS is constantly increasing. High technology treatments are expensive and some of them put a disproportionate cost burden on the NHS. The public now expects that all necessary treatment including the incorporation of major advances in medical science will be provided within the NHS. Resources are never likely to meet this expectation. In such circumstances the doctor should solve his primary problem (of a high expectation from the health services) by explaining the constraints within which he is working to the patient. The problem is on two levels. The first level is the overall funding and that is where politics come in. The second is the point of contact with the patient – where the doctor works with the resources provided.

The process of budgetary allocation is such that within the NHS the budget is allocated to health authorities. Each authority in turn takes professional advice and then the budget is subdivided. Doctors can influence these decisions but lack direct control over them.

Finite resources can never match potentially infinite demands or expectations. The inevitable consequence is that a decision to allocate a particular sum to a particular service will produce underfunding of another service. This will result in a number of possible outcomes (e.g. ward closure/staff reductions/ increased waiting lists) all of which may increase morbidity.

As the resources available within the NHS are limited, the doctor has a general duty to advise on their equitable allocation and efficient use. This duty is, however, subordinate to his professional duty to the individual who seeks his clinical advice. It is the doctor's ethical duty to use the most economic and efficacious treatment available.

It is also the doctor's duty to co-operate with research into the rational use of resources. The doctor should be objective about the allocation of resources and research into resources. However, it is essential that the doctor retains his clinical freedom to act in the patient's best interests.

If conditions are inadequate, nationally or locally, the doctor has a responsibility to warn those responsible of the possible consequences. This obligation is strengthened by the doctor's necessary authority as the person identifiably responsible for managing the patient's illness. If, as a result of resource restriction, the conditions in which a doctor is required to practise fall below the minimum level he finds acceptable, he may feel that it would be unethical to continue to advise and treat patients in a situation where his ability to offer treatment is curtailed.

At local level, resource allocation can mean that the service may be reduced to a point where the doctor has to assess whether he can continue to perform his job. At this level the doctor has the most influence in the process. The doctor is often obliged to decide which patient to treat. The doctor should not hide the need to take such a decision from his patients; to do so would be to revert to paternalism.

Decisions on resource allocation at the level of patient contact can be made according to various criteria. The criteria most often used are medical need, e.g. treating those who are most seriously ill, and welfare maximisation, e.g. treating those who will live longest, or who have the most dependents. Other criteria may be merit, partiality, social or economic worth, cost effectiveness or random selection but these can be discounted easily as unacceptable both logically and morally. In recent years, the decisions required in connection with resource allocation have led to attempts to judge the probability of medical success. This in turn has led health economists to develop the concept of quality adjusted life years (QUALYs) which is a crude indicator of the success of different forms of treatment.

Most doctors choose the criterion of medical need as it is the easiest to apply using clinical judgement. However, problems may arise in choosing between patients whose medical needs are the same.

A problem which frequently confronts the profession is that health authorities cannot always afford an adequate number of professional staff for locum/holiday cover. Even if funds can be found, the cover cannot always be obtained. This means that the remaining staff often work long hours and cannot be at the mental and physical peak required to perform their duties effectively. This problem is faced by all health professionals. If staff resources are inadequate, then the work level should be reduced in order to maintain safe treatment for those patients under care. As a result, waiting lists may grow and doctors may be forced to decide which patients to treat and how to treat them. Thus the doctor may ultimately have to decide on whether a withdrawal of services is appropriate. Doctors hold widely differing views about withdrawal of their services. Where adequate resources necessary for the treatment of patients are not available to the doctor, opinions will differ as to the circumstances which would, if at all, justify such action.

Withdrawal of services from a monopoly employer has much greater consequences for the community than withdrawal of services from a near-monopoly employer or from one of a number of competing employers, since in the former case no alternative exists to provide even an emergency supply. Were an NHS monopoly to exist, doctors could not treat patients outside it and would therefore find themselves totally prevented by their ethical responsibilities from even a temporary withdrawal of services. Such a situation presents the ethical dilemma at its most critical (see: Chapter 15 – Continuing Ethical Dilemmas).

Eventually the doctor may decide to tell the patient that treatment is not available because of lack of funds. The clinical decision to do this is straightforward. Nevertheless, all doctors will be aware that in telling a patient that the State resources are inadequate he is directly criticising the government's budgetary allocation to the health service and that patients may complain to politicians. Such a consideration must not prevent the doctor from explaining the difficulties he is experiencing to his patient.

14 Research

When a doctor encounters patients in the field of medical research, his relationship to them may change in that in some cases there may be no therapeutic benefit to the patient and there may be an element of risk. Nevertheless, the doctor still carries a heavy responsibility for the continued well-being of his patients. The Declaration of Geneva states 'the health of my patient will be my first consideration' and that 'a physician shall only in the patient's interest'. Therefore great care must be taken that the concept of informed consent be followed closely and that the patient understands fully any possible risks or discomfort which might be involved. The patient must be exposed to the minimum of discomfort and danger. It is unethical to conduct research which is badly planned or poorly executed.

The Declaration of Helsinki states that the patient's interest must come first. In certain circumstances, for example where no known treatment for a condition exists, a doctor may know that the proposed treatment for a patient may be unpleasant, uncomfortable and possibly dangerous. The possibility of a cure, however, either for the patient or for future patients, may lead him to consider exposing that patient to the risks and discomfort involved in the hope of some alleviation of the patient's condition. There is a very fine line which must be followed when applying the Declaration of Helsinki to research when the doctor believes that the interests of a particular patient may be subordinated to the greater good of future sufferers. As stated in the Declaration of Helsinki 'the potential subject must be adequately informed of the aims, methods, anticipated benefits and potential hazards of the study and the discomfort it may entail. He or she is at liberty to abstain from participation in the study and he or she is free to withdraw his or her consent to participation at any time'.

The very nature of research yields a possibility that a patient's interests may take second place to a researcher's objectives. Ethical review must always be carefully applied and if it appears that patients are being subjected to unacceptable risk or discomfort in any part of the study, the study must be stopped. There are, of course, some projects which are non-experimental involving, for example, the extensive study of case records. In this case the confidentiality of identifiable information about patients involved must be protected. It is possible to divide research, which involves direct therapeutic interference with a patient, into that which will possibly benefit the individual participant and that which is not likely to do so.

Where the assessment of one treatment against another is being undertaken and it is decided to use a placebo or to conduct a double-blind trial, care must be taken that those patients who are being used as controls are not disadvantaged in any way because they receive either a treatment which is known to be less effective than the best available or no treatment at all. Some form of placebo may be used if there is no known treatment, but if a known therapy is available the best should be used as a control against the new therapy which is being assessed. In other words, patients may be informed that a clinical trial is in progress and that they are being given either the best proven treatment or an unproven alternative which may be better or worse.

In paediatric research there are specific problems which should be considered before the study begins. If the investigation cannot be expected to benefit the individual patient the hazards should be examined carefully and weighed against the benefits for future patients. Although parents can give consent for treatment or indeed research on their children where there is a possibility of therapeutic treatment, where a child understands what is happening then his refusal to co-operate, particularly in painful or uncomfortable research, should be respected (see Ethical Codes and Statements – Helsinki Declaration).

If the subjects of research are in an enclosed or restricted environment the problem of consent is extremely important. For example, in research on prisoners it is possible that a prisoner might expect benefits from agreeing to participate in a research programme though this may not have been stated. All manner of pressures can apply in these circumstances and, therefore, it is unethical to carry out a research procedure on a prisoner that is of no direct benefit to him or her.

In the Armed Forces or indeed in the case of medical students or junior doctors, pressures may be applied to the participants which for various reasons they feel unable to resist. Great care should be taken to make certain that these individuals take part in a research procedure freely and without any pressure. There may be circumstances in which medical students may be exposed to hazards which are unacceptable even if they have given free consent; this must be carefully explored by the Ethical Committee whose permission has been sought.

In occupational medicine, research may be undertaken into the environment or into the hazards of a particular industry for the purpose of statutory investigations.

If foetal material or a foetus are to be used in research, those undertaking the project should read the Report of the Advisory Group on the Use of Foetuses and Foetal Material for Research (HMSO, 1972) and the BMA's Interim Guidelines on the Use of Foetal Tissue in Transplantation Therapy (Appendix III).

There is a recommended Code of Practice (Appendix IV).

In all research projects, an approved ethical committee must be consulted before any research takes place. The BMA has produced guidance on the constitution of ethical committees (see Appendix V). The size of the committee varies from district to district, but non-medical members should always be involved in decisions. Nothing is more calculated to destroy the trust of the public in research than if decisions seem to be made without proper non-medical representation. There may be advantages in the case of multi-centre trials for approval by a national ethical research committee.

In clinical trials on new drugs, great care must be taken not only with the assessment of the ethical committee, but with regard to the advice of the Committee on Safety of Medicines. A Code of Practice for Assessment of Licensed Medicines in General Practice has been published by the ABPI. In future, every protocol sent to a doctor will be accompanied by a copy of the ABPI Code. Financial reward for undertaking clinical trials on behalf of a drug company must be carefully considered; any money received in excess of the expenses of the clerical work or equipment required should be scrutinised with great care having regard to the GMC advice.

15 Continuing Ethical Dilemmas

Advances in medicine and changing patterns of disease alter the nature of some ethical problems and bring others into sharper focus. Medical ethics must also take into account changes in social, cultural and religious values. The quest for permanent, fixed responses to ethical problems is illusory. Movement may be slow and imperceptible but an evolutionary process is nevertheless taking place.

Termination of Pregnancy

The general principles enunciated in the 'Statement on Therapeutic Abortion' by the World Medical Association in 1970, known as the Declaration of Oslo, are broadly applicable to practice in the United Kingdom. However, legislation in different countries varies and the Abortion Act 1967 has created problems for the doctor.

Because risk of injury to the health of a woman is statistically smaller if a pregnancy is terminated in the early months than if it is allowed to go to term, some people argue that abortion is justified if the woman requests it. But she needs a doctor to carry it out and the Act contains a 'conscientious objection' clause by which the doctor can refuse to participate in treatment, though he has a duty to assist the patient to obtain alternative medical advice (and in the case of general practitioners in contract with a Family Practitioner Committee the duty to indicate to the patient alternative sources of advice as part of the contract) if she wants it.

The patient's immediate wishes may conflict with the doctor's judgement of her best long-term interests. If so, the doctor must be prepared to make arrangements for the patient to obtain a second opinion.

If a girl under the age of sixteen requests termination without her parents' knowledge, the doctor may feel conflict between his duty to confidentiality and his responsibilities to the girl's parents or guardian. This cannot be resolved by any rigid code of practice. The doctor should attempt to persuade the girl to allow him to inform her parents or guardian, but what he decides to do will depend upon his judgement of what is in the best interests of the patient.

The Abortion Act 1967 specifically states that 'nothing in the Act shall affect the provisions of the Infant Life (Preservation) Act 1929'. This Act makes reference to a child 'capable of being born alive'. It further states that if a woman has been pregnant for 28 weeks or more it shall be prima facie proof that her child was capable of being born alive. However, it does not state that a child born before 28 weeks is not capable of being born alive and in fact such premature babies have sometimes survived. The doctor should recommend or perform termination after 20 weeks only if he is convinced that the health of the woman is seriously threatened, or if there is good reason to believe that the child will be seriously handicapped. If the doctor is uncertain he should always consult other colleagues and follow his own conscience, all in the best interests of his patient.

Attempts have been made to amend the 1967 legislation, but at the present time 28 weeks remains the official period for legal viability of the foetus.

The Treatment of Sub-Fertility and Infertility

For religious or conscientious reasons, some doctors do not wish to use certain forms of treatment available for sub-fertile couples. However, those doctors have an ethical duty to help such couples arrive at their own ethical decisions without unreasonable intrusion of the doctor's own beliefs. If the doctor cannot provide such help or if the couples wish to seek a form of treatment which the doctor finds unacceptable, he is under an ethical obligation to ensure that the couple are referred to a medical practitioner who does provide treatment.

Artificial Insemination by Donor Semen

The doctor has an ethical duty to consider the circumstances, in so far as they can be foreseen, of the child born as a result of successful inseminations. He must be satisfied that those concerned have considered the implications including the possibility of some genetic or other defect in the semen and the resultant handicap in the child.

Because of the genetic implications of one donor becoming responsible for large numbers of offspring, the remote risk of related offspring marrying one another must be considered. The Warnock Committee concluded that this risk would remain remote if such treatment took place only at registered centres with an absolute limit of ten successful inseminations per donor. The BMA fully endorses this conclusion.

The doctor has an ethical responsibility to assess the effect of the procedure upon the dynamics of the family. The child has a claim on a normal family life but the stresses resulting from the subfertility together with the stresses inherent in the procedure itself may seriously prejudice the family relationships. The doctor should explore with the couple, both separately and together, their understanding of the procedure and their attitudes towards it. Only when he is satisfied that the various issues have been fully explained, and when he believes that the relationship is likely to remain stable, is it ethical for the doctor to proceed.

The British Medical Association supports efforts to secure a change in the law, so that a child born as a result of AID, to which the husband of the mother has consented in writing, is recognised as legitimate from the time of confirmation of conception.

Genetic Counselling and Investigation

The patient's right to autonomy in genetic counselling and research may be in conflict with the need for other affected individuals to have access to such information. Certainty about an individual's genotype might affect his attitudes to life, and society's attitudes to him with the possibility of considerable medical, economic and social repercussions. A patient may be found to be carrying an abnormal gene but may be reluctant to allow this knowledge to be given to other family members. Is the individual entitled to total autonomy or, because of the shared nature of genetic material, does the information belong to all members of the family who may wish to take preventive measures for themselves in the light of the information? On balance, the importance of such information outweighs the importance of complete medical confidentiality. The information should be kept confidential to the medical profession and to those entitled to it because of their potential carrier state. A carrier's spouse or potential spouse should be told because they may bear some responsibility for passing on such genes to future generations.

Tissue and Organ Transplantation

Codes covering investigative and surgical procedures provide adequate safeguards for live adult donors. Written consent should be obtained from the donor after a full explanation of the procedure involved and the possible consequences to him. The donor may also be advised to discuss the procedure with relatives, religious advisers, or anyone close to the patient and these advisers should be able to meet the doctors if they wish. The General Medical Council, in its Annual Report of 1985, stated that:

> '. . . it is unethical and improper for a registered medical practitioner, wittingly or unwittingly, to encourage or take part in any way in the development of such trafficking in the sale of human organs; and that, accordingly, no surgeon should undertake the transplantation of a non-regenerative organ from a living donor without first making due inquiry to establish beyond reasonable doubt that the donor's consent has not been given as a result of any form of undue influence'.

There are probably no circumstances in which a child can be considered a suitable donor of non-regenerative tissue. There is considerable legal doubt about a parent's right to give consent on behalf of the child, but even if this exists that right cannot extend to any procedure which is not in the child's best interests.

81

Bone marrow transplantation is an example of the donation of regenerative material. In many cases, tissue compatibility and the natural history of the disease means that the only suitable donor will be a child. In cases where a doctor considers the discomfort to a donor is minimal it is ethical to perform a bone marrow transplant with the consent of the parent. The procedure can be handled ethically only in the context of a compassionate and objective assessment of the individuals and families concerned and the doctor must weigh up carefully the risk for the donor in reaching his final decision. It is unethical to transplant tissues from a donor without personally assuring that he is not carrying antibodies of HIV.

For the transplant of unpaired organs, the only possible donor is a dead person. Death may be certified after brain death and the decision that brain death has occurred. The criteria relating to the certificates of brain death are laid out in paragraphs 28–30 of the Code of Practice 'Cadaveric Organs for Transplantation' and must be followed (HMSO, 1983).

Jehovah's Witnesses and Blood Transfusion

When a Jehovah's Witness is suffering a condition for which the normal treatment may involve blood transfusion, the doctor should advise the patient of this. If, as is probable, the patient refuses to consent to transfusion, the doctor must decide whether this caveat greatly increases the risk of the procedure. He must then reassess whether the risk from the disease outweighs the risk of the treatment without the ability to transfuse blood. The doctor may decide not to continue either because he believes that the possible benefits are outweighed by the potential dangers of the treatment, or because he is unwilling to have his options for management curtailed. If he declines further treatment for the latter reason he must make every effort to refer the patient to a colleague who would be willing to undertake the case.

If the doctor decides to proceed with the treatment he must honour his undertaking to the patient having fully explained his concern about the results of withholding any part of the treatment.

When the child of a Jehovah's Witness requires a transfusion the doctor may feel that the child should be made a ward of court or, if time does not allow, the doctor may proceed with the transfusion having the written agreement of a colleague supporting his opinion that the transfusion is necessary. The situation of the unborn child requiring an in utero transfusion remains unresolved.

Transplantation of foetal tissue

Anticipating the potential use of foetal material for transplant purposes, the Central Ethical Committee of the BMA drew up an interim statement endorsed by BMA Council, 1988 entitled 'Interim Guidelines on the Use of Foetal Tissue in Transplantation Therapy' (Appendix III).

16 Continuing Ethical Dilemmas – No Consensus View

In Vitro Fertilisation

The techniques now exist to fertilise ova and sperm in vitro from sub-fertile couples' donor sperm, donor ova and from both donor sperm and donor ova. Many children have now been born using each of these methods. The ability to fertilise ova outside the womb raises considerable ethical and moral issues. The BMA endorses the Warnock Committee's conclusions that all these techniques are ethically acceptable providing that certain safeguards exist. These include a clear definition of the legal status of the resulting child. The doctor has an ethical obligation to the unborn child as well as to the parents who consult him. Centres where such techniques are carried out should be registered and subject to legislative control. In the meantime, the BMA welcomes the present voluntary regulatory code.

It is ethically acceptable for experiments to be conducted on unwanted gametes up to fourteen days before their destruction and disposal, in order to improve existing techniques, to improve success rates and reduce unnecessary interference with patients. The profession is divided on the question of whether embryos should be created especially for the purpose of research. Research into appropriate storage of gametes and of fertilised ova will continue to be required, including the most appropriate external media for the fertilisation and storage process.

Like members of the Warnock Committee, the profession is also divided on ethically acceptable research involving manipulation within the fertilised ovum. This development, which paves the way for genetic engineering, will have profound long-term ethical consequences. Such research is ethically acceptable only when it has a direct and immediate clinical purpose. General research with no clearly defined objective is unethical. It is unethical for a doctor to be associated directly or indirectly with any procedures involving fertilisation between human and non-human gametes even though the resulting conceptus will be immediately destroyed.

Surrogacy

Under the Surrogacy Arrangements Act 1985 the recruitment of surrogate mothers for financial gain is illegal. Proposed amendments to this Act would render criminal the activities of a surrogate mother and commissioning parents and those professionals, including doctors, who knowingly assist in establishing a surrogate pregnancy whether or not in a commercial context. In 1985, however, the BMA resolved 'that this Meeting agrees with the principle of surrogate births in selected cases with careful controls'.

In considering his involvement in a non-commercial surrogate pregnancy, the doctor has an equal ethical obligation to the child as to his patient. The child's status will at best be ambiguous. Both natural and commissioning parents may disown the child. It is widely agreed that all children now have a right to know their origins. The doctor should be satisfied that the commissioning parents are genuinely and permanently infertile and that no other treatment offers any prospect of relief. As far as the doctor is able to determine they must be able to provide a normal family home. So homosexual couples and single parents are excluded. The doctor is under an ethical obligation to undertake thorough screening of the surrogate mother and he must be satisfied that no covert financial arrangements exist. These restrictions will inevitably make the conditions in which a surrogate pregnancy is ethically acceptable very exceptional.

All doctors have an ethical responsibility to come to the aid of a pregnant woman who seeks their help and provide for such a mother the maximum help consistent with the doctor's training and experience, irrespective of how the pregnancy was conceived.

Severely Malformed Infants

A malformed infant has the same rights as a normal infant. It follows that ordinary non-medical care which is necessary for the maintenance of the life of a normal infant should not be withheld from a malformed infant.

Where medical or surgical procedures might be needed to preserve the life of a severely malformed infant every opportunity should be taken for deliberation and discussion as time permits. The closest possible co-operation between the doctor in charge, the parents of the child and any colleagues whose opinions are felt to be helpful, including the patient's general practitioner, is essential. The doctor has a particular duty to ensure the parents have as full an understanding as possible of the options and the likely outcome with or without surgery or other means of active intervention.

The parents of an infant born severely malformed must never be left with the feeling that they are having to exercise their responsibility to make decisions regarding consent to the management of their child without help and understanding. They should be encouraged to seek advice from anyone in whose judgement they have faith. The doctor in charge is responsible for the initiation or the withholding of treatment in the best interests of the child. He must attend primarily to the needs and rights of the child but he must also have concern for the family as a whole.

If doubt persists in the minds either of the parents or the doctor in charge as to the best interests of the infant, a second medical opinion should be sought.

In emergencies there may be no time for consultation with parents or anyone else and the doctor in charge must exercise his clinical judgement.

Screening for Disease

There are many different definitions of screening; this section concerns a variety of ethical dilemmas which arise from the discovery of a potential disease process at a stage before the patient would present to the doctor with signs or symptoms of the disease. The dilemmas arising from screening have common features no matter how the patient becomes involved in the screening process. The process is initiated by the doctor or the health service rather than by a patient. Alternatively the individual may seek a particular screening procedure. In the latter he does so either because the service has been offered to him or because he believes such a service should be offered to him. This change in the traditional mode of presentation implies that the doctor has a benefit to offer. Should any harm result from the screening procedure, such as the incorrect labelling of a fit person as diseased, the doctor cannot claim that he was merely responding as best he could to the patient's distress and request for help. Furthermore, a screening procedure is not necessarily diagnostic in itself. Almost invariably it will fail to identify some individuals who are at risk and who are then given unjustified reassurance, and it will also identify some individuals who are not at risk but who are thereby disadvantaged by the unexpected (and unjustified) 'discovery'.

Screening in Epidemics

As part of measures to control an outbreak of infectious disease, it may be appropriate to test contacts of the index case for the presence of micro-organisms. Such a procedure may identify the origin of the outbreak and the extent of its spread beyond the index case. Such procedures may involve cases or carriers discovered by the screening process. Unless some positive action will be undertaken as a result of the screening process which will have a direct benefit to the community as a whole, it is almost certainly unethical to undertake such screening. Furthermore, a consequence of a positive finding may be temporary restriction of the individual's liberty. The critical ethical factors must therefore be the severity of the disease and the risk of spread within the rest of the community as a whole.

Health Risks in Industry

In the food industry, screening of prospective employees is a preventive measure against the spread of food-borne disease. Under statute, typhoid carriers may be permanently excluded from any involvement in the food industry. In a wide variety of other industries screening of prospective employees is undertaken either to protect the employee from harm within the industry or to protect the community from risk resulting from such an employee. These forms of screening are ethically acceptable subject to the general reservations expressed above and subject to the nature, purpose and significance of the tests being explained to the employee as part of the employment application process. If a prospective employee is rejected as a result of these screening tests, the nature of the results and their significance should be explained to him. Where appropriate, arrangements should be made for referral to his usual medical attendant.

Screening Services

The NHS and a number of commercial organisations offer a variety of screening services directly to the public. Although the decision to be screened is taken by the individual there is a general expectation that the service is reliable, and that it will accurately identify problems for which some preventive or therapeutic remedy exists. These expectations cannot always be realised. In participating in such services, doctors must be satisfied that the balance of advantage for the potential patient lies in undergoing the test and that some positive action will be taken in the light of the results obtained. In the absence of either of these requirements, it is probably unethical to proceed.

Doctor-Initiated Screening for Diagnostic Purposes

An increasing number of diagnostic tests are used by doctors to discover rare and unlikely alternatives to the presumptive diagnosis and to establish certain levels of fitness to undertake the therapeutic procedure, e.g. haemoglobin level, where surgery is contemplated. Such screening tests are clearly ethical because they are an essential part of the original medical consultation.

The increasing sophistication of laboratory analytic equipment enables a wide range of other investigations to be performed on the same sample at the same time at no extra cost. Indeed, it may be more expensive to exclude such investigations. Ethical difficulties may, however, arise if any of these unsolicited tests prove to be positive. In these circumstances the doctor must explain the implications of the findings to the patient and make adequate arrangements for their further investigation and, if appropriate, treatment.

Screening for Research Purposes

The remains of samples obtained for clinical purposes are frequently stored, often for long periods. These samples are used for quality testing in the laboratory and for developing and validating new tests. Where samples have been stored for long periods they may be used to assess the incidence of conditions for which no suitable laboratory test existed at the time the sample was taken. Samples may be used as part of a research project into medical conditions which have apparently become more or less common over time. It has to be recognised that by its very nature, random screening of this kind precludes any identification or tracking back to identify a positive result obtained from a sample in this anonymous way from a particular district or clinic.

Acquired Immune Deficiency Syndrome

The disease now widely known as AIDS is presenting major ethical dilemmas as individual communities seek to grapple with the apparent significance of its current spread. The lack of any therapeutic remedy, its continuing advance and its high rate of fatality have deep implications for society. In such an atmosphere, it is easy for community leaders and doctors to conclude that the need to control the spread of the disease justifies almost any means of potential control. The medical profession must review the developing pattern of the disease and evaluate each new proposal against the ethical judgements discussed in this Handbook.

Although the virus (HIV) is infectious, its infectivity appears to be relatively low. It is certain types of intimate sexual contact and the use of infected needles, largely by drug abusers, and transfusion of infected blood which offer any major risk of spread. The condition is therefore in effect a sexually transmitted disease in which the principles of autonomy have traditionally outweighed the wider needs of the community (Venereal Diseases Act 1917). It is part of the duty of doctors to allay exaggerated fears among the general public about the spread of the disease from normal sexual contact which could result in pregnancy, having regard to the advice available from various sources and the normal duties of selected groups, e.g. police.

It should be remembered that the disease is not unique in its characteristics. Other diseases such as hepatitis B are spread in similar ways, are considerably more infectious and are a greater hazard to health care workers, even though the risk of death from this disease is minimal compared to that of dying from AIDS. Protection against the theoretical risk of transmission to health care workers is simple and effective. It is unethical for a doctor to withhold care from a patient who is or whom he suspects to be HIV positive. It is unreasonable and unethical to insist that a patient should be screened to identify the level of risk to health care workers.

Experience of the condition is providing information which may be useful to HIV carriers in delaying the onset of evident disease. For the foreseeable future, preventive strategies offer the only practical response to the disease. The strategies raise a variety of ethical dilemmas. There is some debate as to whether the 'safe sex' campaigns reduce casual sexual relationships. Equally, vigorous messages dealing with all other risk factors (not only sexual) are being actively promoted. The problems posed by AIDS add a new dimension to the problems associated with early sexual relationships and the contraceptive advice which should be given to younger patients.

Testing for HIV antibody is now compulsory for those offering to donate blood or tissue. Testing is available to all those who request it although it is now strongly recommended that individuals should be counselled before submitting specimens for this purpose. Routine testing of pregnant women is being encouraged and some would argue that it should be compulsory. For many years women have been routinely screened during pregnancy for syphilis in order that prompt treatment may be given to both mother and child. Knowledge of the mother's HIV status will not safeguard her baby since no effective treatment is available and the outcome is currently universally bad. If screening is undertaken early in pregnancy, preferably before the eighteenth week at the latest, it could be of value to the mother since immediate termination would reduce her risk of early onset of the disease. Screening of blood specimens taken for other purposes would provide additional evidence about the spread of the virus in the general population. Such screening would be ethical only if the specimens were made anonymous as described in an earlier section with no possibility of tracing back to an individual.

The final ethical issue concerns the confidentiality of HIV status. There is a benefit to doctors and nurses in being aware of a particular patient's antibody status. In practice, though, it is extremely difficult to restrict the disclosure of such information only to those who 'need to know'. There have been virtually no problems with the implementation of the NHS Venereal Diseases Regulations 1974 or the preceding legislation in the field. Individuals should be encouraged to disclose this information to their dental and nursing attendants but in the final analysis must have the right to refuse disclosure.

This issue is also extended by the requests from insurance companies for general practitioners to provide information about patients who are seeking insurance. General practitioners should complete insurance company forms truthfully to the best of their knowledge, but should make it clear to the patient what information is being disclosed, and what the possible implications may be. It is then up to the patient to decide whether the form should be sent. Attempts by insurance companies to obtain unsubstantiated information from doctors may well lead patients to conceal worries about the risk of HIV infection, and enlarge the pool of undetected HIV carriers. General practitioners should not make statements about their patients' lifestyles unless they are absolutely certain of the facts. For example, a patient should never be described as a homosexual or possibly homosexual unless he has himself told his doctor of this. Otherwise, the general practitioner should say that he does not know any relevant lifestyle details.

There is strong pressure outside the profession for AIDS to be made statutorily notifiable. There are also demands for information about antibody status within the population to be made more widely known. The system developed by the Communicable Disease Surveillance Centre ensures that the necessary information is available to those who need it while preserving the patient's right to confidentiality to date, and should continue to safeguard this in relation to

AIDS. Community physicians have powers under the Public Health Acts to control the liberty of AIDS patients whose infectious state is a serious risk to the community. Wider disclosure would have profound ethical, social and political consequences which are not justified by the present stage of development of the disease.

The Doctor and the Dying Patient

When a doctor's relationship is with a patient not capable of being cured and who is approaching death, ethical problems have to be faced. This is the area where the interface between medical ethics and society's ethics is most common. It is also the area where the rules are hardest to apply; no single answer will fit all situations. The doctor's primary aim to ensure the well-being of his patient is unchanged and that includes the stages when recovery is not possible. The doctor should aim to ensure that his patient dies with dignity and as little suffering as possible.

In the course of a prolonged terminal illness the relationship between doctor and patient may become close and much discussion may take place with an opportunity to talk over the basic issues dealt with in this section. Naturally this also applies to the caring relatives. During these discussions the doctor may develop an understanding of how much or how little the patient and his caring relatives wish to have done as death approaches.

The ability to maintain artificially 'physiological life' while a patient remains unconscious, dependent on machines for long periods of time, complicates the issue further. Clearly the sustaining of physiological functions with no prospect of recovery of consciousness or contact with the patient's environment has led to considerable debate as to whether or not such support should be continued. There is also debate as to who should be responsible for making the decisions to keep the systems working or not. Some believe that doctors must always preserve life for as long as possible; others feel that such support should only occasionally be continued for any significant time. There is no rigid code by which such decisions can be made; it is up to each doctor in this situation to examine the case with reference to his own ethical viewpoint, the wishes of the relatives and, if possible, to find out what the patient's own views are on the subject beforehand.

There are patients being maintained on systems who are in fact 'brain dead'. In October 1976 the Conference of Medical Royal Colleges and their Faculties in the United Kingdom published a report expressing the opinion that this could be diagnosed with uncertainty. A subsequent report by the Conference of 15 January 1979 concluded that the identification of brain death means that the patient is dead whether or not the functions of some organs such as a heart beat are still being maintained by artificial means. Termination of the support system therefore does not cause the patient's death and brings no ethical problems.

Euthanasia

Whilst the title of this section remains 'euthanasia', it should be noted that the BMA Working Party on euthanasia recommended that this term be no longer used because of the many interpretations this word has been given, including those set out below. The Working Party advocates the use of the terms 'active intervention to shorten life' and 'non-treatment decisions' which reflect more accurately the areas of concern.

When a patient is not being maintained on a support system, but is incurable and in severe pain or distress, the question of euthanasia arises. The word means literally 'gentle and easy death' but has come to be interpreted by some as 'mercy killing' involving a direct deliberate single act or series of acts. Within the literal meaning of the word there are no ethical difficulties for the doctor. As stated above he has responsibility to ensure that his patient dies with dignity and as little suffering as possible. The concept of 'mercy killing' must be further explored and has been further modified by the application of the words 'compulsory', 'voluntary', 'active' and 'passive' to euthanasia. In no country is euthanasia yet legal. Bills legalising voluntary euthanasia were defeated in Parliament in 1936, 1969 and 1976.

Note must be taken of the recent trends in the Netherlands. There, if a doctor agrees to help a patient die and goes through a set of procedures involving consultation with the patient, the relatives and colleagues, then it is unlikely that doctor will be prosecuted under Dutch law. This is a new situation and will need evaluation when it has been working for some time.

Compulsory euthanasia – meaning a decision by society that an individual either against his will or without being able to consent should have his life terminated – is totally abhorrent to the medical profession. Voluntary euthanasia – in which an individual, either in advance by means of a so-called 'living will', or at the time but in full control of his faculties, expresses a wish that in certain circumstances his life should be terminated – does have followers and there are associations for its promotion. What then is the prevailing view of the profession?

In 1971 the BMA undertook a major review of euthanasia. The 1971 report concluded:

> 'Euthanasia cannot be accepted by the medical profession; in rejecting it doctors will be supported by the majority of laymen who share the belief that the deliberate killing of a helpless person can never be condoned. It is right that dying patients should be relieved of suffering and this can and should be done. Killing patients is no part of the work of doctors and nurses';

And the European Convention of Human Rights says:

> 'Everyone's right to life shall be protected by law. No one shall be deprived of life intentionally save in the execution of a sentence of a court following his conviction of a crime for which this penalty is provided by law'.

Policy dating from 1971 was recently reviewed by a Working Party which reported to Council in May 1988. Its conclusions are as follows:

1. Some patients see death as the fitting conclusion to the events of their life. These people may wish neither to hasten their death nor to delay it. For them, death is a mystery which they approach with tranquillity. There are limits to medical science and it is inappropriate for doctors to insist on intruding in these circumstances.

2. There is a distinction between an active intervention by a doctor to terminate life and a decision not to prolong the life (a non-treatment decision). In both of these categories there are occasions on which a patient will ask for one of these courses of action to be taken and times when the patient could say but does not. There are also occasions where the patient is incompetent to decide.

3. An active intervention by anybody to terminate another person's life should remain illegal. Neither doctors nor any other occupational group should be placed in a category which lessens their responsibility for their actions.

4. In clinical practice there are many cases where it is right that a doctor should accede to a request not to prolong the life of a patient. Appropriate medical skills and techniques should be offered to patients when there is a good chance of providing an extension of life that will have the quality that the patient seeks.

5. Patient autonomy is a crucial aspect of informed patient care. This is achieved most successfully where a trusting and open relationship between the doctor and the patient allows participation in decisions about illness and its treatment. Doctors should regard patients as authorising treatment, and should respect those authorisations and any decision to withdraw consent. But autonomy works both ways. Patients have the right to decline treatment but do not have the right to demand treatment which the doctor cannot, in conscience, provide. An active intervention by a doctor to terminate a patient's life is just such a 'treatment'. Patients cannot and should not be able to *require* their doctors to collaborate in their death. If a patient does make such a request there should be a presumption that the doctor will not agree.

6. More important than debate about the limits of autonomy is the need for doctors and everyone else who is involved in the care of the terminally ill, to communicate with their dying patients. Doctors need to be able to elicit the fears of dying patients and to discuss and answer those fears. They need to be able to discuss terminal care openly so that patients see that they will not be abandoned and left helpless in the face of a terminal disease. Only if such communication and good treatment becomes the norm can society expect to dissipate the pressure to force doctors to do things that the medical profession should not accept.

7. The killing of an individual who is certain to suffer severe pain, and to be isolated from human warmth and compassion as they die, is held by some to be very similar to the situation of the terminally ill patient. In the hypothetical case of the person trapped in a hotel fire there may appear to be no alternative to a decision to intervene actively to end the person's life. This applies equally to the actions of army doctors in Burma in the second world war. Today, however, terminal medical care is offered by individuals and groups dedicated to the relief of suffering and respect for the feelings and worth of the dying patient. These aims are achieved regularly and with considerable success. The two situations are not comparable.

8. Requests from young and severely disabled patients for a doctor's intervention to end their life present one of the hardest problems in day to day care. Counselling is essential to reaffirm the value of the person, and to counter pressure which may be created by the feeling of being unloved and an embarrassment or inconvenience to those upon whom the patient is wholly dependent. The subtle and dynamic factors surrounding disability and the wish to die make any drastic change in the law unwise for this group of patients.

9. Any move toward liberalising the active termination of a severely malformed infant's life would herald a serious and incalculable change in the present ethos of medicine. Nevertheless, there are circumstances where the doctor may judge correctly that continuing to treat an infant is cruel and that the doctor should ease the baby's dying rather than prolong it by the insensitive use of medical technology.

10. This kind of decision requires careful communication between doctor, parents, nursing staff and other care-givers. It is imperative that the doctor should start from a position which seeks to preserve and value life rather than, on occasion, to judge it as not worthwhile. It is important also to stress that withholding treatment does not preclude loving care for the dying infant. This will, of course, involve relieving the infant's distress.

11. An overwhelming majority of those who are rescued from serious suicide attempts do not repeat their attempts. This means that individuals who make such a choice about their own deaths do not always affirm this in the light of reflection. The techniques developed in the Netherlands mean that the opportunity for reflection is unlikely to be available to a person when a doctor acts to terminate their life.

12. Advance declarations of the type envisaged are not yet recognised as binding by English or, we believe, Scottish law. They may be a valuable guide to the wishes of a patient who can no longer participate in clinical decisions, but should not be regarded as immutable or legally binding prescriptions for medical care. They require respectful attention and sensitive interpretation.

13. The law's deep seated adherence to intent rather than consequence alone is an important reference point in the moral assessment of any action. A decision to withdraw treatment which has become a burden and is no longer of continuing benefit to a patient, has a different intent to one which involves ending the life of a person. We accept drug treatment which may involve a risk to the patient's life if the sole intention is to relieve illness, pain, distress or suffering.

14. Any doctor, compelled by conscience to intervene to end a person's life, will do so prepared to face the closest scrutiny of this action that the law might wish to make.

15. The law should not be changed and the deliberate taking of a human life should remain a crime. This rejection of a change in the law to permit doctors to intervene to end a person's life is not just a subordination of individual well-being to social policy. It is, instead, an affirmation of the supreme value of the individual, no matter how worthless and hopeless that individual may feel.

Withdrawal of Services

The vocation to heal and care for the sick is implicit in taking up the practice of medicine and for centuries the withholding from the sick of medical skills possessed by a physician was unthinkable. However, with changes in organised society in the 20th century, doctors, who are increasingly being employed as salaried workers with clearly defined contracts and conditions of work, find themselves in conflict with their employers either about working conditions, adequate resources for safe health care or remuneration.

This has been so serious on a number of occasions, that the doctors have had to consider withdrawal of services from organised systems of health care in order to achieve the necessary changes. This situation is not limited to doctors in salaried positions.

The general principle when withholding such services takes place has been that an 'emergency' service should be provided for the duration of the action; thus life-threatening illness requiring immediate action to preserve life has been covered by the emergency doctors.

However, this does not guarantee that all suffering is treated. Furthermore, it means that treatment of such conditions as cancers may be delayed as they may not constitute an immediate emergency. This may lead to a shortened life expectancy. There is no doubt that such action would increase human suffering.

This poses the question as to how far the medical profession can withhold its services to achieve changes, and what minimum emergency services are compatible with professional ethical standards – indeed, whether a 'strike' is ever ethically acceptable. The moral and ethical questions need to be considered in relation to the propriety of taking industrial action at all.

It is clear that since the 19th century, when governmental socially-organised medical care developed and with the huge increase in salaried rather than free practising doctors in the 20th century, considerable new problems have arisen for the moral and ethical aspects of medical care. This is made worse with increased social security involvement in health care and collective agreements between the profession and social security (often governmental) organisations.

Mention has been made about the rights of patients. In considering industrial action the human rights of doctors also have to be considered and the individual and collective responsibilities of doctors must be explored.

A physician's entitlement, in common with all other citizens, to the fundamental right to withhold his labour is clearly tempered by the responsibilities which he accepts when he enters the medical profession.

Broadly these constitute the duty to use his skills to cure or to ease suffering and to ensure that, should he withdraw from treatment, continuity of care is safeguarded.

Effectively this means that a total strike or withdrawal of labour is ethically unacceptable. However, this does not preclude industrial action such as non-participation in administration of the Health Care Services or limited withdrawal of labour, subject to the provisions mentioned above.

In an NHS where much practice can be performed only in facilities belonging to the NHS such as hospitals and operating theatres such activity is the most difficult as physicians may find themselves unable to offer the necessary services outside the system. They therefore have a duty, if they are in conflict with a near-monopoly employer either over resources for care or poor working conditions, to ensure that in the event of withdrawal, adequate arrangement is made for treating emergencies and the continuing care of those already undergoing treatment.

Ethical Codes and Statements

The Hippocratic Oath

The methods and details of medical practice change with the passage of time and the advance of knowledge. However, many fundamental principles of professional behaviour have remained unaltered through the recorded history of medicine. The Hippocratic Oath was probably written in the 5th century BC and was intended to be affirmed by each doctor on entry to the medical profession. In translation it reads as follows:

> I swear by Apollo the physician, and Aesculapius and Health, and All-heal, and all the gods and goddesses, that, according to my ability and judgement, I will keep this Oath and this stipulation – to reckon him who taught me this Art equally dear to me as my parents, to share my substance with him, and relieve his necessities if required; to look upon his offspring in the same footing as my own brothers, and to teach them this Art, if they shall wish to learn it, without fee or stipulation; and that by precept, lecture and every other mode of instruction, I will impart a knowledge of the Art to my own sons, and those of my teachers, and to disciples bound by a stipulation and oath according to the law of medicine, but to none other. I will follow that system of regimen which, according to my ability and judgement, I consider for the benefit of my patients, and abstain from whatever is deleterious and mischievous. I will give no deadly medicine to anyone if asked, nor suggest any such counsel; and in like manner I will not give to a woman a pessary to produce abortion. With purity and with holiness I will pass my life and practise my Art. I will not cut persons labouring under the stone, but will leave this to be done by men who are practitioners of this work. Into whatever houses I enter, I will go into them for the benefit of the sick, and will abstain from every voluntary act of mischief and corruption; and, further, from the seduction of females, or males, of freemen or slaves. Whatever, in connection with my professional practice, or not in connection with it, I see or hear, in the life of men, which ought not to be spoken of abroad, I will not divulge, as reckoning that all such should be kept secret. While I continue to keep this Oath unviolated, may it be granted

to me to enjoy life and the practice of the Art, respected by all men, in all times. But should I trespass and violate this Oath, may the reverse be my lot.

The World Medical Association

The BMA was a founder member of the WMA and remained a member until January 1984. The statements which follow fall into 2 categories. Those which were adopted during the period of BMA membership with their full co-operation and those which have subsequently been adopted by the WMA, without BMA involvement.

The following declarations have been drawn up from time to time by the World Medical Association and have been endorsed by the BMA.

International Code of Medical Ethics

One of the first acts of the World Medical Association, when formed in 1947, was to produce a modern restatement of the Hippocratic Oath, known as the Declaration of Geneva, and to base upon it an International Code of Medical Ethics which applies in times of both peace and war. The Declaration of Geneva, as amended by the 22nd World Medical Assembly, Sydney, Australia, in August 1968 and the 35th World Medical Assembly, Venice, Italy, in October 1983, reads:

At the time of being admitted as a member of the Medical Profession:

I solemnly pledge myself to consecrate my life to the service of humanity;

I will give to my teachers the respect and gratitude which is their due;

I will practise my profession with conscience and dignity;

The health of my patient will be my first consideration;

I will respect the secrets which are confided in me, even after the patient has died;

I will maintain by all the means in my power, the honour and the noble traditions of the medical profession;

My colleagues will be my brothers;

I will not permit considerations of religion, nationality, race, party politics or social standing to intervene between my duty and my patients;

I will maintain the utmost respect for human life from its beginning even under threat and I will not use my medical knowledge contrary to the laws of humanity;

I make these promises solemnly, freely and upon my honour.

The English text of the International Code of Medical Ethics is as follows:

Duties of physicians in general

A PHYSICIAN SHALL always maintain the highest standards of professional conduct.

A PHYSICIAN SHALL not permit motives of profit to influence the free and independent exercise of professional judgement on behalf of patients.

A PHYSICIAN SHALL, in all types of medical practice, be dedicated to providing competent medical service in full technical and moral independence, with compassion and respect for human dignity.

A PHYSICIAN SHALL deal honestly with patients and colleagues, and strive to expose those physicians deficient in character or competence, or who engage in fraud or deception.

The following practices are deemed to be unethical conduct:

(a) Self advertising by physicians, unless permitted by the laws of the country and the Code of Ethics of the National Medical Association.

(b) Paying or receiving any fee or any other consideration solely to procure the referral of a patient or for prescribing or referring a patient to any source.

A PHYSICIAN SHALL respect the rights of patients, of colleagues, and of other health professionals, and shall safeguard patient confidences.

A PHYSICIAN SHALL act only in the patient's interest when providing medical care which might have the effect of weakening the physical and mental condition of the patient.

A PHYSICIAN SHALL use great caution in divulging discoveries or new techniques or treatment through non-professional channels.

A PHYSICIAN SHALL certify only that which he has personally verified.

Duties of physicians to the sick

A PHYSICIAN SHALL always bear in mind the obligation of preserving human life.

A PHYSICIAN SHALL owe his patients complete loyalty and all the resources of his science. Whenever an examination or treatment is beyond the physician's capacity he should summon another physician who has the necessary ability.

A PHYSICIAN SHALL preserve absolute confidentiality on all he knows about his patient even after the patient has died.

A PHYSICIAN SHALL give emergency care as a humanitarian duty unless he is assured that others are willing and able to give such care.

Duties of physicians to each other

A PHYSICIAN SHALL behave towards his colleagues as he would have them behave towards him.

A PHYSICIAN SHALL NOT entice patients from his colleagues.

A PHYSICIAN SHALL observe the principles of 'The Declaration of Geneva' approved by the World Medical Association.

Subsequently, the World Medical Association has considered and published material on a number of ethical matters.

Discrimination in medicine

The following motion on the subject of discrimination in medicine was adopted by the World Medical Association in 1973:

> WHEREAS: The Declaration of Geneva, adopted and published by the World Medical Association, states, *inter alia*, that, 'I (a medical practitioner) WILL NOT PERMIT considerations of religion, nationality, race, party politics or social standing to intervene between my duty and my patient';
>
> THEREFORE, BE IT RESOLVED by the 27th World Medical Assembly meeting in Munich, that the World Medical Association *vehemently condemns* colour, political and religious discrimination of any form in the training of medical practitioners and in the practice of medicine and in the provision of health services for the peoples of the world.

Rights of the patient

In 1981 the World Medical Association adopted a Statement on the rights of the patient. Known as the Declaration of Lisbon, it reads:

> Recognising that there may be practical, ethical or legal difficulties, a physician should always act according to his/her conscience and always in the best interest of the patient. The following Declaration represents some of the principal rights which the medical profession seeks to provide to patients.
>
> Whenever legislation or government action denies these rights of the patient, physicians should seek by appropriate means to assure or to restore them.
>
> (a) The patient has the right to choose his physician freely.
>
> (b) The patient has the right to be cared for by a physician who is free to make clinical and ethical judgements without any outside interference.
>
> (c) The patient has the right to accept or to refuse treatment after receiving adequate information.

(d) The patient has the right to expect that his physician will respect the confidential nature of all his medical and personal details.

(e) The patient has the right to die in dignity.

(f) The patient has the right to receive or to decline spiritual and moral comfort including the help of a minister of an appropriate religion.

Human experimentation

In 1964, the World Medical Association drew up a code of ethics on human experimentation. This code, known as the Declaration of Helsinki, as amended by the 29th World Medical Assembly, Helsinki, Finland, in 1975, and by the 35th World Medical Assembly, Venice, Italy, in 1983, reads:

It is the mission of the medical doctor to safeguard the health of the people. His or her knowledge and conscience are dedicated to the fulfilment of this mission.

The Declaration of Geneva of the World Medical Association binds the physician with the words, 'The health of my patient will be my first consideration', and the International Code of Medical Ethics declares that 'A physician shall act only in the patient's interest when providing medical care which might have the effect of weakening the physical and mental condition of the patient'.

The purpose of biomedical research involving human subjects must be to improve diagnostic, therapeutic and prophylactic procedures and the understanding of the aetiology and pathogenesis of disease.

In current medical practice most diagnostic, therapeutic or prophylactic procedures involve hazards. This applies especially to biomedical research.

Medical progress is based on research which ultimately must rest in part on experimentation involving human subjects.

In the field of biomedical research a fundamental distinction must be recognised between medical research in which the aim is essentially diagnostic or therapeutic for a patient, and medical research, the essential object of which is purely scientific and without implying direct diagnostic or therapeutic value to the person subjected to the research.

Special caution must be exercised in the conduct of research which may affect the environment, and the welfare of animals used for research must be respected.

Because it is essential that the results of laboratory experiments be applied to human beings to further scientific knowledge and to help suffering humanity, the World Medical Association has prepared the following recommendations as a guide to every physician in biomedical research involving human subjects. They should be kept under review in the future. It must be stressed that the standards as drafted are only a guide to physicians all over the world. Physicians are not relieved from criminal, civil and ethical responsibilities under the laws of their own countries.

I Basic principles

1. Biomedical research involving human subjects must conform to generally accepted scientific principles and should be based on adequately performed laboratory and animal experimentation and on a thorough knowledge of the scientific literature.

2. The design and performance of each experimental procedure involving human subjects should be clearly formulated in an experimental protocol which should be transmitted to a specially appointed independent committee for consideration, comment and guidance.

3. Biomedical research involving human subjects should be conducted only by scientifically qualified persons and under the supervision of a clinically competent medical person. The responsibility for the human subject must always rest with the medically qualified person and never rest on the subject of the research, even though the subject has given his or her consent.

4. Biomedical research involving human subjects cannot legitimately be carried out unless the importance of the objective is in proportion to the inherent risk to the subject.

5. Every biomedical research project involving human subjects should be preceded by careful assessment of predictable risks in comparison with foreseeable benefits to the subject or to others. Concern for the interests of the subject must always prevail over the interest of science and society.

6. The right of the research subject to safeguard his or her integrity must always be respected. Every precaution should be taken to respect the privacy of the subject and to minimize the impact of the study on the subject's physical and mental integrity and on the personality of the subject.

7. Physicians should abstain from engaging in research projects involving human subjects unless they are satisfied that the hazards involved are believed to be predictable. Physicians should cease any investigation if the hazards are found to outweigh the potential benefits.

8. In publication of the results of his or her research, the physician is obliged to preserve the accuracy of the results. Reports of experimentation not in accordance with the principles laid down in this Declaration should not be accepted for publication.

9. In any research on human beings, each potential subject must be adequately informed of the aims, methods, anticipated benefits and potential hazards of the study and the discomfort it may entail. He or she should be informed that he or she is at liberty to abstain from participation in the study and that he or she is free to withdraw his or her consent to participation at any time. The physician should then obtain the subject's freely-given informed consent, preferably in writing.

10. When obtaining informed consent for the research project the physician should be particularly cautious if the subject is in a dependent relationship to him or her or may consent under duress. In that case the informed consent should be obtained by a physician who is not engaged in the investigation and who is completely independent of this official relationship.

11. In case of legal incompetence, informed consent should be obtained from the legal guardian in accordance with national legislation. Where physical or mental incapacity makes it impossible to obtain informed consent, or when the subject is a minor, permission from the responsible relative replaces that of the subject in accordance with national legislation. Whenever the minor child is in fact able to give a consent, the minor's consent must be obtained in addition to the consent of the minor's legal guardian.

12. The research protocol should always contain a statement of the ethical considerations involved and should indicate that the principles enunciated in the present Declaration are complied with.

II Medical research combined with professional care (Clinical research)

1. In the treatment of the sick person, the physician must be free to use a new diagnostic and therapeutic measure, if in his or her judgement it offers hope of saving life, re-establishing health or alleviating suffering.

2. The potential benefits, hazards and discomfort of a new method should be weighed against the advantages of the best current diagnostic and therapeutic methods.

3. In any medical study, every patient – including those of a control group, if any – should be assured of the best proven diagnostic and therapeutic method.

4. The refusal of the patient to participate in a study must never interfere with the physician-patient relationship.

5. If the physician considers it essential not to obtain informed consent, the specific reasons for this proposal should be stated in the experimental protocol for transmission to the independent committee (I.2).

6. The physician can combine medical research with professional care, the objective being the acquisition of new medical knowledge, only to the extent that medical research is justified by its potential diagnostic or therapeutic value for the patient.

III Non-therapeutic biomedical research involving human subjects (Non-clinical biomedical research)

1. In the purely scientific application of medical research carried out on a human being, it is the duty of the physician to remain the protector of the life and health of that person on whom biomedical research is being carried out.

2. The subjects should be volunteers – either healthy persons or patients for whom the experimental design is not related to the patient's illness.

3. The investigator or the investigating team should discontinue the research if in his/her or their judgement it may, if continued, be harmful to the individual.

4. In research on man, the interest of science and society should never take precedence over considerations related to the well-being of the subject.

Therapeutic abortion

In 1970 the World Medical Association drew up a Statement on Therapeutic Abortion. This code, known as the Declaration of Oslo, was amended by the 35th World Medical Assembly, Venice, Italy, in October 1983, and states.

1. The first moral principle imposed upon the physician is respect for human life from its beginning.

2. Circumstances which bring the vital interests of a mother into conflict with the vital interests of her unborn child create a dilemma and raise the question whether or not the pregnancy should be deliberately terminated.

3. Diversity of response to this situation results from the diversity of attitudes towards the life of the unborn child. This is a matter of individual conviction and conscience which must be respected.

4. It is not the role of the medical profession to determine the attitudes and rules of any particular state or community in this matter, but it is our duty to attempt both to ensure the protection of our patients and to safeguard the rights of the physician within society.

5. Therefore, where the law allows therapeutic abortion to be performed, the procedure should be performed by a physician competent to do so in premises approved by the appropriate authority.

102

6. If the physician considers that his convictions do not allow him to advise or perform an abortion, he may withdraw while ensuring the continuity of (medical) care by a qualified colleague.

7. This statement, while it is endorsed by the General Assembly of the World Medical Association, is not to be regarded as binding on any individual member association unless it is adopted by that member association.

Medical secrecy

The following Resolution on 'Medical secrecy' was adopted by the World Medical Association in 1973:

WHEREAS: The privacy of the individual is highly prized in most societies and widely accepted as a civil right; and

WHEREAS: The confidential nature of the patient-doctor relationship is regarded by most doctors as extremely important and is taken for granted by the patient; and

WHEREAS: There is an increasing tendency towards an intrusion on medical secrecy;

THEREFORE BE IT RESOLVED that the 27th World Medical Assembly reaffirm the vital importance of maintaining medical secrecy not as a privilege for the doctor, but to protect the privacy of the individual as the basis for the confidential relationship between the patient and his doctor; and ask the United Nations, representing the people of the world, to give to the medical profession the needed help and to show ways for securing this fundamental right for the individual human being.

Use of computers in medicine

The following statement, adopted by the World Medical Assembly in 1973, was amended by the 35th World Medical Assembly in Venice, Italy, in October 1983, and reads:

The World Medical Association, having taken note of the great advances and advantages resulting from the use of computers and electronic data processing in the field of health, especially in patient care and epidemiology, makes the following recommendations:

1. National medical associations should take all possible steps to ensure the privacy, the security and confidentiality of information on their patients;

2. It is not a breach of confidentiality to release or transfer confidential health care information required for the purpose of conducting scientific research, management audits, financial audits, program

evaluations, or similar studies, provided the information released does not identify, directly or indirectly, any individual patient in any report of such research, audit or evaluation, or otherwise disclose patient identities in any manner;

3. National medical associations should oppose any effort to enact legislation on electronic data processing which could endanger or undermine the right of the patient to privacy, security and confidentiality. Effective safeguards against unauthorised use or retransmission of social security numbers and other personal information must be assured before such information enters the computer;

4. Medical data banks should never be linked to other central data banks.

Torture and other cruel, inhuman or degrading treatment or punishment

In 1975 the World Medical Association adopted the following guidelines for medical doctors concerning Torture and Other Cruel, Inhuman or Degrading Treatment or Punishment in relation to Detention and Imprisonment (Declaration of Tokyo):

Preamble

It is the privilege of the medical doctor to practise medicine in the service of humanity, to preserve and restore bodily and mental health without distinction as to persons, to comfort and to ease the suffering of his or her patients. The utmost respect for human life is to be maintained even under threat, and no use made of any medical knowledge contrary to the laws of humanity.

For the purpose of this Declaration, torture is defined as the deliberate, systematic or wanton infliction of physical or mental suffering by one or more persons acting alone or on the orders of any authority, to force another person to yield information, to make a confession, or for any other reason.

Declaration

1. The doctor shall not countenance, condone or participate in the practice of torture or other forms of cruel, inhuman or degrading procedures, whatever the offence of which the victim of such procedures is suspected, accused or guilty, and whatever the victim's belief or motives, and in all situations, including armed conflict and civil strife.

2. The doctor shall not provide any premises, instruments, substances or knowledge to facilitate the practice of torture or other forms of

cruel, inhuman or degrading treatment or to diminish the ability of the victim to resist such treatment.

3. The doctor shall not be present during any procedure during which torture or other forms of cruel, inhuman or degrading treatment is used or threatened.

4. A doctor must have complete clinical independence in deciding upon the care of a person for whom he or she is medically responsible. The doctor's fundamental role is to alleviate the distress of his or her fellow men, and no motive, whether personal, collective or political, shall prevail against this higher purpose.

5. Where a prisoner refuses nourishment and is considered by the doctor as capable of forming an unimpaired and rational judgement concerning the consequences of such a voluntary refusal of nourishment, he or she shall not be fed artificially. The decision as to the capacity of the prisoner to form such a judgement should be confirmed by at least one other independent doctor. The consequences or the refusal of nourishment shall be explained by the doctor or the prisoner.

6. The World Medical Association will support, and should encourage the international community, the national medical association and fellow doctors, to support the doctor and his or her family in the face of threats or reprisals resulting from a refusal to condone the use of torture or other forms of cruel, inhuman or degrading treatment.

Terminal illness

In 1983 the World Medical Association adopted a statement on Terminal illness (Declaration of Venice), which reads:

1. The duty of the physician is to heal and, where possible, relieve suffering and act to protect the best interests of his patients.

2. There shall be no exception to this principle even in the case of incurable disease or malformation.

3. This principle does not preclude application of the following rules:

   3.1 The physician may relieve suffering of a terminally ill patient by withholding treatment with the consent of the patient or his immediate family if unable to express his will. Withholding of treatment does not free the physician from his obligation to assist the dying person and give him the necessary medicaments to mitigate the terminal phase of his illness.

   3.2 The physician shall refrain from employing any extraordinary means which would prove of no benefit for the patient.

3.3 The physician may, when the patient cannot reverse the final process of cessation of vital functions, apply such artificial means as are necessary to keep organs active for transplantation provided he acts in accordance with the laws of the country or by virtue of a formal consent given by the responsible person and provided the certification of death or the irreversibility of vital activity had been made by physicians unconnected with the transplantation and the patient receiving treatment. These artificial means shall not be paid for by the donor or his relatives. Physicians treating the donor shall be totally independent of those treating the recipient and of the recipient himself.

Statements on Death

World Medical Association

The World Medical Association formulated a Statement on Death in 1968. Known as the Declaration of Sydney, it was amended by the 35th World Medical Assembly in Venice, Italy, in 1983, and reads:

1. The determination of the time of death is in most countries the legal responsibility of the physician and should remain so. Usually the physician will be able without special assistance to decide that a person is dead, employing the classical criteria known to all physicians.

2. Two modern practices in medicine, however, have made it necessary to study the question of the time of death further:

    (a) the ability to maintain by artificial means the circulation of oxygenated blood through tissues of the body which may have been irreversibly injured and

    (b) the use of cadaver organs such as heart or kidneys for transplantation.

3. A complication is that death is a gradual process at the cellular level with tissues varying in their ability to withstand deprivation of oxygen. But clinical interest lies not in the state of preservation of isolated cells but in the fate of a person. Here the point of death of the different cells and organs is not so important as the certainty that the process has become irreversible by whatever techniques of resuscitation that may be employed.

4. It is essential to determine the irreversible cessation of all functions of the entire brain, including the brain stem. This determination will be based on clinical judgement supplemented if necessary by a number of diagnostic aids. However, no single technological criterion is entirely satisfactory in the present state of medicine nor can any one technological procedure be substituted for the overall judgement of

the physician. If transplantation of an organ is involved, the decision that death exists should be made by two or more physicians and the physicians determining the moment of death should in no way be immediately concerned with the performance of the transplantation.

5. Determination of the point of death of the person makes it ethically permissible to cease attempts at resuscitation and, in countries where the law permits, to remove organs from the cadaver provided that prevailing legal requirements of consent have been fulfilled.

Conference of Medical Royal Colleges

The following Memorandum was issued by the Honorary Secretary of the Conference of Medical Royal Colleges and their Faculties in the United Kingdom on 15 January 1979:

1. In October 1976 the Conference of Royal Colleges and their Faculties (UK) published a report unanimously expressing the opinion that 'brain death', when it had occurred, could be diagnosed with certainty. The report has been widely accepted. The conference was not at that time asked whether or not it believed that death itself should be presumed to occur when brain death takes place or whether it would come to some other conclusion. The present report examines this point and should be considered as an addendum to the original report.

2. Exceptionally, as a result of massive trauma, death occurs instantaneously or near-instantaneously. Far more commonly, death is not an event: it is a process, the various organs and systems supporting the continuation of life failing and eventually ceasing altogether to function, successively and at different times.

3. Cessation of respiration and cessation of the heart beat are examples of organic failure occurring during the process of dying, and since the moment that the heart beat ceases is usually detectable with simplicity by no more than clinical means, it has for many centuries been accepted as the moment of death itself, without any serious attempt being made to assess the validity of this assumption.

4. It is now universally accepted, by the lay public as well as by the medical profession, that it is not possible to equate death itself with the cessation of the heart beat. Quite apart from the elective cardiac arrest of open-heart surgery, spontaneous cardiac arrest followed by successful resuscitation is today a commonplace, and although the more sensational accounts of occurrences of this kind still refer to the patient being 'dead' until restoration of the heart beat, the use of the quote marks usually demonstrates that this word is not to be taken literally, for to most people the one aspect of death that is beyond debate is its irreversibility.

5. In the majority of cases in which a dying patient passes through the processes leading to the irreversible state we call death, successive organic failures eventually reach a point at which brain death occurs and this is the point of no return.

6. In a minority of cases brain death does not occur as a result of the failure of other organs or systems but as a direct result of severe damage to the brain itself from, perhaps, a head injury or a spontaneous intracranial haemorrhage. Here the order of events is reversed; instead of the failure of such vital functions as heart beat and respiration eventually resulting in brain death, brain death results in the cessation of spontaneous respiration; this is normally followed within minutes by cardiac arrest due to hypoxia. If, however, oxygenation is maintained by artificial ventilation the heart beat can continue for some days, and haemoperfusion will for a time be adequate to maintain function in other organs, such as the liver and kidneys.

7. Whatever the mode of its production, brain death represents the stage at which a patient becomes truly dead, because by then all functions of the brain have permanently and irreversibly ceased. It is not difficult or illogical in any way to equate this with the concept in many religions of the departure of the spirit from the body.

8. In the majority of cases, since brain death is part of or the culmination of a failure of all vital functions, there is no necessity for a doctor specifically to identify brain death individually before concluding that the patient is dead. In a minority of cases in which it is brain death that causes failure of other organs and systems, the fact that these systems can be artificially maintained even after brain death has made it important to establish a diagnostic routine which will identify with certainty the existence of brain death.

Conclusion

9. It is the conclusion of the Conference that the identification of brain death means that the patient is dead, whether or not the function of some organs, such as heart beat, is still maintained by artificial means.

The Commonwealth Medical Association

The following Ethical Code of the Commonwealth Medical Association was approved at its meeting in Jamaica in 1974:

1. The doctor's primary loyalty is to his patient.

2. His vocation and skill shall be devoted to the amelioration of symptoms, the cure of illness and the promotion of health.

3. He shall respect human life and studiously avoid doing it injury.

4. He shall share all the knowledge he may have gained with his colleagues without any reserve.

5. He shall respect the confidence of his patient as he would his own.

6. He shall by precept and example maintain the dignity and ideals of the profession, and permit no bias based on race, creed or socio-economic factors to affect his professional practice.

Note: The word 'patient' used in this Code embraces the prisoner or other persons whom a doctor might be called upon to attend at another's bidding.

Standing Committee of Doctors of the EC

The Standing Committee of Doctors of the EC adopted the following Declaration concerning the practice of medicine within the Community at its Plenary Assembly Session held in Nuremburg in November 1967 (Charter of Nuremburg (orig. French)). The text is as published in *The Handbook of Policy Statements 1959–1982*, Standing Committee of Doctors of the EC.

1. Every man must be free to choose his doctor. Every man must be guaranteed that whatever a doctor's obligations vis-a-vis society, whatever he confides to his doctor and to those assisting him will remain secret.

   Every man must have a guarantee that the doctor he consults is morally and technically totally independent and that he has free choice of therapy.

   Human life from its beginning and the human person in its integrity, both material and spiritual, must be the object of total respect.

   Guarantees of these rights for patients imply a health policy resulting from firm agreement between those responsible to the state and the organised medical profession.

2. The aim common to the health policy of states and medical practice is to protect the health of all its citizens.

   It is the duty of states to take all precautions to ensure all social classes – without discrimination – have access to all the medical care they require. Every man has the right to obtain from the social institutions and the medical corps the help he needs to preserve, develop or recover his health: he has an obligation to contribute materially and morally to these objectives.

   Economic expansion finds one of its principal human justifications in the advancement of resources allocated to health; the medical profession intends to do all in its power to increase, at equal costs, the human and social effectiveness of medicine.

3. The unusual necessary contact between the doctor and his patient takes account of the fact that these two partners belong to one community, a condition of all health and social policy. But there must be reciprocal confidence between the patient and his doctor based on the certitude that in his treatment the doctor holds in the highest esteem and has consciously consecrated all his knowledge to the service of the human person. No matter what his method of practice or remuneration the doctor must have access to the existing resources necessary for medical intervention; he must have free choice of decision bearing in mind the interests of his patient and the concrete possibilities offered by the advancements of science and medical techniques.

    Doctors must be free to organise their practice together in a manner complying with the technical and social need of the profession, on condition that moral and technical independence be respected and the personal responsibility of each practitioner maintained.

4. Whatever its method of practice the medical profession is one. These methods are complementary. They derive from the same deontology although they may be submitted to different organisation conditions. Respect for moral laws and for the basic principles of medical practice is assured by independent institutions, emanating from the medical corps and invested, particularly under the highest judicial processes in the country, with disciplinary and judicial power.

    Every doctor has a moral obligation to actively participate in his professional organisation. Through this organisation he participates in the elaboration of the country's health policy. Members of the profession can and must fight for respect of basic principles in the practice of medicine, on condition that the rights of the patient are safeguarded.

5. Hospital equipment must be within the compass of its specific mission in the service of the whole population. Its establishment is the result of a planned policy in which the public powers and the organised profession participate, allocating to public power and private initiative fuller distribution of health establishments. It comprises a variety of establishments, graded and co-ordinated among themselves, meeting the task or several tasks given to it: prevention, care, rehabilitation, teaching, research. . . . This organisation as a whole must take into consideration the principles given in the hospital charter drawn up by the Standing Committee of Doctors of the EC and respect the autonomy of each establishment which must entail administrative and medical direction. The professional independence of the hospital doctor must be

guaranteed by unquestionable criteria of nomination and a statute assuring him stability of function, economic independence and social protection.

'Technical progress, the basis of our industrial civilisation, and economic expansion which is its fruit, have for their natural end, especially thanks to a health policy, to bring about full physical and spiritual development of man, of all men'.

European Union of General Practitioners (UEMO)

The European Union of General Practitioners (UEMO) adopted the following statement on Medical Confidentiality in Relation to the use of Modern Methods of Communication (EDP) in Medicine at Amsterdam in May 1979:

The patient has a right to expect that his doctor will maintain professional confidentiality towards third parties.

When modern methods of communications are employed, therefore, which for medical, scientific or administrative reasons involve the recording of data in such a way that they no longer remain under the direct control of the doctor, it is necessary to take all possible security measures to ensure the maintenance of confidentiality.

Under the pretext of better planning of health policy, of scientific research based on more reliable statistics, of more rapid access to medical records in case of accident and of general rationalisation for the sake of efficiency, efforts are being made to gather together in data banks large amounts of information on individual patients. This involves the danger that these data will be recorded, examined and transmitted by third parties without the possibility of the patient concerned or his doctor judging the necessity for such actions or of monitoring the nature, the importance and the use of these data in individual cases.

General practitioners believe that personal data received by the doctor in the course of his professional duties should be released to a computerised data system accessible to third parties other than surgery or hospital staff, only when the following safeguards are applied:

1. The permission of both the patient and his doctor should have been obtained.

2. The patient should be able to obtain information on the nature and the implications of the data recorded about him, but that such information should only be transmitted through the doctor who supplied the data or, where appropriate, the doctor who is treating him.

3. The patient in agreement with his doctor, should be able to correct or delete information appearing on the record.

4. Safeguards should be applied to prevent abuse of the information or access by unauthorised persons.

5. All personal information of a medical nature should be kept separate from other types of information accessible to persons other than the doctor.

6. That the responsibility for the use of computerised medical data-systems should rest exclusively with doctors.

The European Union of General Practitioners (UEMO) emphasises that all legislation should take into account the principles and conditions laid down above.

Appendix I

BRITISH MEDICAL ASSOCIATION

Inter Professional Working Group on Access to Personal Health Information

Subject: **Statement on Subject Access to Personal Health Information**
Approved: **BMA Council 5 3 86**
Reference: **British Medical Journal, 1983, 286, 1592**

We support the right of patients and clients to have access to all information which is held about them on their behalf. Such access encourages openness and can improve the quality of the record by correcting factual errors and reducing misunderstandings. However, there are some situations in which the un-regulated release of the entire clinical or social record could cause distress, or even harm, to a patient or client, or to someone else. In some cases, the personal record may also include information on others who are entitled to have their confidences kept. Also, many records would be unintelligible to a layman without professional interpretation and explanation.

For all these reasons, the imposition of an *absolute* requirement to afford unrestricted access could inhibit health professionals from recording sensitive information or opinions to the inevitable detriment of patient care: an acceptable mechanism must therefore be devised for the exercise of a proper discretion by the responsible clinician or other health professional. This should provide for subject access to the extent and in the manner judged most helpful by the responsible clinician or an appropriate colleague. Any subject who is dissatisfied with this arrangement should then have a right to seek access through an independent health professional of his choice, practising in the same discipline or specialty as the responsible clinician or other health professionals. There may, in the last resort, remain a legal right to seek access to information which has still been withheld. It would be appropriate for such a right to be exercised through the courts, which could decide the issue. We believe that this would arise only exceptionally.

We shall deal in a separate statement with access to personal health information records by third parties other than the patient or client.

Appendix II

Guidelines for Doctors and Nurses Who Have Been Asked to Help in Connection with the Implementation of Section 55 of the Police and Criminal Evidence Act 1984 (Intimate Searches)

General

These guidelines have been drawn up in collaboration with the Royal College of Nursing and are intended to help doctors and nurses make a decision as to whether or not to comply with a request from the police to conduct an intimate search in connection with Section 55 of the Police and Criminal Evidence Act 1984.

Section 55 of the Act states that:

'55 –(1) Subject to the following provisions of this section, if an officer of at least the rank of superintendent has reasonable grounds for believing –

(a) that a person who has been arrested and is in police detention may have concealed on him anything which –
  (i)   he could use to cause physical injury to himself or others; and
  (ii) he might so use while he is in police detention or in the custody of a court, or
(b) that such a person –
  (i)   may have a Class A drug concealed on him; and
  (ii) was in possession of it with the appropriate criminal intent before his arrest, he may authorise such a search of that person . . .'

The Act states that an officer may not authorise an intimate search of a suspect for anything unless he has reasonable grounds for believing that it cannot be found without the suspect being intimately searched. However, the health professional must also satisfy himself that the police have such reasonable grounds. He should therefore ask the police for details of the evidence which they believe gives them grounds for suspicion and form his own opinion of it. If the health professional is not satisfied with this evidence he should refuse to perform an intimate search.

The authorisation to conduct an intimate search must be made, according to the law, by an officer of at least the rank of superintendent although the law provides for a chief inspector to do this on occasion. He may make the authorisation either orally or in writing. We would normally expect this authorisation to have been made in writing and produced to the health professional. However, this may not be possible in unusual or urgent circumstances. If the authorisation has been made orally the police officer making the authorisation should speak directly to the doctor. A written copy of the authorisation should be sent to the doctor as soon as possible.

We have established a hierarchy of health professionals whom the police will contact in order to find someone to perform the search. This is as follows:

1. A police surgeon

2. Another registered medical practitioner

3. A registered midwife

4. A registered nurse

The RCN has advised that nurses should only conduct intimate searches if the only alternative person to carry out a search is a police officer.

The Intimate Search

Acquiescence

In the surroundings of the police station where a refusal to perform an intimate search may imply guilt, it is very unlikely that the health professional will be able to obtain freely the consent of the suspect to perform an intimate search. However, except on very rare occasions, an intimate search should not be performed without the subject's acquiescence having been obtained first. This should be in written form and should have been obtained after the doctor has had the opportunity to talk to the suspect on his own.

Whereabouts

The Police and Criminal Evidence Act states that an intimate search in connection with a possible drug offence may not be carried out at a police station but permits other intimate searches to be carried out at the police station. Nevertheless, we believe that all intimate searches should be conducted either at hospital, at a registered medical practitioner's surgery or at some other premises used for the delivery of health care. There may be rare exceptions to this rule where an immediate search is necessary.

Grounds

Section 55 distinguishes between the two main reasons why a police officer may request an intimate search. Section 55(1)(a) allows a search if the suspect is believed to have concealed upon him an object which he could use to cause physical injury to himself or to others and Section 55(1)(b) deals with the suspected concealment of Class A drugs. The ethical issues raised by these two sub-sections are substantially different and so have been dealt with separately below.

Grounds for a search under Section 55(1)(a)

There is no objection to carrying out an intimate body search when the purpose is to remove an object which is of immediate danger to the life or personal safety of those people responsible for the suspect's custody and supervision or other people. It is in these circumstances only that it may be necessary to carry out the search at a police station and without the subject's acquiescence.

We are not convinced that there are sufficient grounds for an intimate search if a non-acquiescing suspect is believed to have concealed upon him an object or substance which will not harm others but only himself. He should have the risks he may be taking fully explained to him. If the health professional is satisfied that the suspect understands the risk and the suspect still refuses a search, the health professional should not perform a search except under very exceptional circumstances.

The police have a reserve power to carry out an intimate search under this section.

Grounds for a search under Section 55(1)(b)

It may also be permissible to carry out a search for heroin if there is absolutely no alternative. The 'reserve powers' of the police which allow them to carry out intimate searches do not apply in connection with drug offences. The health professional should therefore take great care to ensure for himself that the police have taken all other possible action before requesting an intimate search for a drug offence. If he is not satisfied then he should not perform a search.

Non-contact means of searching

The police may, under certain circumstances, detain a suspect in custody for up to 96 hours by applying for warrants for further detention. Unless there are compelling reasons to do otherwise, the health professional should take advantage of this interval. During that time, there may be clear clinical evidence that the suspect is concealing an object. This would render an intimate search unnecessary.

We support the principle that non-contact means of searching should be used where possible. However, the use of the techniques presents problems.

Both x-ray and CT scanning involve radiating the patient. The health professional must therefore have the acquiescence of the patient before undertaking these techniques so that accusations of unnecessary exposure to radiation are avoided. These techniques are not suitable for pregnant women or for one potentially pregnant as at present in the UK abdominal x-ray examinations are not normally carried out in the second half of the menstrual cycle in case conception has occurred. We understand that a popular method of concealing drugs whilst passing through customs is to place approximately 4 grams of a drug in a condom and swallow it.

Although a large number of the grape-sized packets may be swallowed they may well not show up on x-ray or on a CT scan and it may be necessary to ask the suspect to drink a contrast medium in order to outline them. Even so, it may not be possible to distinguish them from ingested food.

Ultrasound is the most suitable technique for non-contact searching and it can demonstrate masses of small density, eg, in the vagina. However, it requires the full co-operation of the patient as, for instance, it is necessary to have a full bladder for a successful examination.

We understand that the very new technique of magnetic resonance would show up small objects. However, this technique is very expensive and only available at a few centres. It is thought that the technique does not have side-effects.

Appendix III

Interim Guidelines on the Use of Foetal Tissue in Transplantation Therapy

The Association has become aware that a number of research centres are developing therapeutic techniques involving the transplantation of foetal tissue, for treatment of conditions including Parkinson's Disease. Such work has now commenced with the recommendations of the Peel Committee on The Use of Fetuses and Fetal Material for Research (1972).

Guidelines

1. Tissue may be obtained only from dead foetuses resulting from therapeutic or spontaneous abortion. Death of the foetus is defined as an irreversible loss of function of the organism as a whole.

2. United Kingdom laws on transplantation must be followed. The woman from whom the foetal material is obtained must consent to the use of the foetal material for research and/or therapeutic purposes.

3. Transplantation activity must not interfere with the method of performing abortions, nor the timing of abortions, or influence the routine abortion procedure of the hospital in any way. Abortions must be performed subject to the Abortion Act, and any subsequent amendments thereof, uninfluenced by the fate of the foetal tissue. The anonymity of the donor should be maintained.

4. The generation or termination of a pregnancy solely to produce suitable material is unethical. There should be no link between the donor and recipient.

5. There must be no financial reward for the donation of foetal material or a foetus.

6. Nervous tissue may only be used as isolated neurones or tissue fragments for transplantation. Other foetal organs may be used as either complete or partial organs for transplantation.

7. All hospital staff directly involved in the procedures – including the abortion – must be informed about the procedures involved.

8. Every project involving transplantation of foetal tissue must be approved by the local ethical research committee.

Appendix IV

Investigation into Foetal Material

DHSS Home and Health Department Working Party – 1972

This code has no binding force, but is the result of careful consideration of all relevant factors in the light of the available evidence. It is hoped that it will prove acceptable to the bodies statutorily responsible for disciplinary matters in the medical and nursing professions.

1. Where a foetus is viable after separation from the mother it is unethical to carry out any experiments on it which are inconsistent with treatment necessary to promote life.

2. The minimal limit of viability for human foetuses should be regarded as twenty weeks' gestational age. This corresponds to a weight of approximately 400–500 grammes.

3. The use of the whole dead foetus or tissues from dead foetuses for medical research is permissible subject to the following conditions.

    (i) The provisions of the Human Tissue Act are observed where applicable;

    (ii) Where the provisions of the Human Tissue Act do not apply there is no known objection on the part of the parent who had an opportunity to declare any wishes about the disposal of the foetus;

    (iii) Dissection of the dead foetus or experiments on the foetus or foetal material do not occur in the operating theatre or place of delivery;

    (iv) There is no monetary exchange for foetuses or foetal material;

    (v) Full records are kept by the relevant institution.

4. The use of the whole pre-viable foetus is permissible provided that:

    (i) The only conditions in paragraph 3 above are observed;

    (ii) Only foetuses weighing less than 300 grammes are used;

(iii) The responsibility for deciding that the foetus is in a category which may be used for this type of research rests with the medical attendants at its birth and never with the intending research worker;

(iv) Such research is only carried out in departments directly related to a hospital and with direct sanction of its ethical committee;

(v) Before permitting such research the ethical committee satisfies itself:

(a) on the validity of the research;

(b) that the required information cannot be obtained in any other way;

(c) that the investigators have the necessary facilities and skill.

5. It is unethical to administer drugs or carry out any procedures during pregnancy with the deliberate intent of ascertaining the harm that they might do the foetus.

Appendix V

BRITISH MEDICAL ASSOCIATION

Central Ethical Committee

Subject: Improving the Network of Local Ethical Research
             Committees and the Establishment of a National
             Ethical Research Committee.

Approved: Council, 8 1 86

Introduction

The Central Ethical Committee's work on improving the network of local ethical research committees began in 1980 when the Committee contacted 138 local ethical research committees and analysed their composition. The analysis showed that there was no set pattern of membership of the Committees and that whilst some were working successfully, others were ineffective. The CEC made suggestions for improving the system and published a paper on local ethical research committees which was approved by BMA Council on 4 March 1981 (BMJ vol 282, 21 March 1981).

By the end of 1983, it was clear that no uniform action had been taken as a result of the BMA's 1981 report. Continued anxieties were being expressed about the ethics of medical research trials and over the effectiveness of local committees. In the meantime, the Inter Professional Working Group on Access to Personal Health Information which was set up to advise government about data protection legislation had confirmed the need for an effective network of local ethical research committees and identified a need for a further committee at national level. These ideas formed the basis of a further policy paper which was approved by BMA Council on 4 January 1984 and which is attached as Appendix I to this document (BMJ 31 March 1984 Annual Report of Council paras 38.19 – 38.21).

In order to stimulate action, the Central Ethical Committee used its 1984 paper as a basis for discussions with the Department of Health and Social Security. The Committee hoped that the DHSS would look into the effectiveness of local committees and reinforce their circular (1974) entitled Supervision of the

Ethics of Clinical Research Investigations and Foetal Research (HSC(IS)153). This circular had advisory status only.

The DHSS was reluctant to take action on this matter which it felt was primarily the concern of the health profession. The Central Ethical Committee has therefore held a series of informal discussions with the interested professional bodies to canvass opinion and establish the extent of common ground within the medical allied professions. Meetings have taken place with representatives of the Royal College of Nursing, the Royal College of Midwives, the Office of Population Censuses and Surveys, the British Psychological Society, the Health Visitors' Association, the British Association of Social Workers, the Council for Professions Supplementary to Medicine and the Committee of Vice Chancellors and Principals. Discussions have also taken place with the Association of Community Health Councils in England and Wales, the Society of Community Health Council Secretaries and Patients' Association. The Conference of Medical Royal Colleges and their Faculties and the Medical Research Council have been kept informed of progress made.

As a result of the various discussions with the interested parties, the Central Ethical Committee has been able to formulate a policy which it believes will be generally acceptable.

Future Arrangements for Local Ethical Research Committees

It is unanimously agreed that an adequate system of local ethical research committees (LERCs) is required to protect and reassure the public and individual patients* (see end). An important, but subsidiary, consideration is that of the protection of the good name of the medical and allied professions, and of individual doctors against, for example, litigation.

Whilst it was suggested by one organisation that a research protocol should be submitted to a two stage evaluation for its scientific merits and then for ethical approval, the general consensus was that it was neither necessary nor desirable to separate these two elements.

The medical profession should recognise the increasing amounts of research undertaken by the paramedical and allied professions. Ethical committees should be so constituted as to take account of this development and so that those with specific professional expertise are consulted when research proposals are considered. There was general agreement that this should be done at local level by a panel of named referees who must be consulted over projects affecting their area of expertise.

One of the problems with local ethical research committees which was identified by nearly all the bodies consulted with was the limitations of their remit. There was general agreement that it was desirable that local ethical

*Clinical research in the context of ethical research committeess embraces any project involving the use of clinical techniques or treatments or the use of personal information about patients.

research committees should be district-based and should be serviced by the District Health Authority. These Committees would be empowered to deal with all clinical research within the district including that undertaken by university departments. It was thought important that academic staff should be *seen* to be dealt with on the same basis as within the NHS. This argument also applied to research in the private sector. Although Family Practitioner Committees are now independent, it was thought equally desirable that research undertaken by general practitioners should be considered by the same district based committee as other clinical research. The problem of lack of co-terminosity of District Health Authority and Family Practitioner Committee boundaries was not insuperable. However, it was recognised that the government may need to make some change to statutory arrangements to allow for general practice research to be considered by a District Health Authority Committee.

It was generally accepted that there should be some sort of appeal system against the decisions of a local ethical research committee. The solution which found most favour was that the researcher should have the right of appeal to two neighbouring local ethical research committees. By this means, there would always be at the very least a majority verdict.

All the bodies consulted were in general agreement that the 1984 policy on local ethical research committees as supplemented by the above was acceptable.

The CEC's new proposals are summarised as follows:

1. Local ethical research committees should be set up by and serviced by District Health Authorities where they do not already exist.

2. They should deal with all clinical research proposals within their geographical area whether from hospital practice, general practice, private practice, universities or industry. Proposals for multi-centre or nation wide research should be handled by the national committee.

3. The membership of the LERC should be:-

2 senior hospital doctors	– nominated by the hospital subcommittee of the District Advisory Committee or equivalent;
1 doctor	– nominated by the board or other responsible committee of the appropriate university;
1 junior hospital doctor	– nominated by the junior medical staff;
2 principals in general practice	– nominated by the LMC after consultation with the local RCGP Faculty;
1 representative of Community Medicine and Community Health	– nominated by the appropriate community medicine and health staff;
1 nurse	– nominated by the DNO or equivalent;
2 lay members	– one nominated by DHSS and one by the CHC but not necessarily from their own membership.

The quorum for meetings should be six people including one lay member.

4. Local ethical research committees must have a panel of referees from the allied professions to whom all research proposals affecting their area of expertise must be referred to discussion by the committee.

5. Advice should be sought from LMCs when statistical information provided by FPCs is released.

6. The remit of local ethical research committees should not preclude them from consultation with any appropriate body.

7. Only in exceptional circumstances should research proposals be vetted by correspondence.

8. Appeals against the decision of a local ethical research committee should be referred to two neighbouring committees.

9. A list of decisions should be available on enquiry and an Annual Report should be prepared.

A National Ethical Research Committee

All the parties consulted agreed about the need to set up a national ethical research committee. It is thought that such a committee should facilitate rather than hinder the consideration of research proposals.

At the present time, any researcher who wishes to undertake research in more than one centre is faced with consulting numerous local ethical research committees. It is thought that a national ethical research committee should consider multi-centre or national level trials and thus speed up the process. This would have the advantage of ensuring consistency in approach and would also save bodies such as the Medical Research Council from being forced to act as their own judge and jury, e.g. in the multi-vitamin trial for spina bifida babies. This will reassure the public.

Teaching centres tend to have a concentration of expertise on abstruse areas of research. An effective method of disseminating this wisdom to local ethical research committees is needed and this should be one of the primary functions of a national ethical research committee. Equally, it is desirable to have a mechanism which can sift and hold a library of good practice filtering up from the LERCs. Thus, a national ethical research committee could act as a central reference committee and disseminate information upon request to local ethical research committees. In addition, the national ethical research committee should draw up its own guidance but this would only be disseminated to local ethical research committees upon request.

All parties agreed that it was of the utmost importance not to undermine the position of LERCs. Nor should researchers be encouraged to refer up to the national ethical research committee proposals other than those which were multi-centre or nationally based. It was for this reason that the idea of using the national ethical research committee as an appellate body was rejected.

Membership of the National Ethical Research Committee

As one of the primary functions of the national ethical research committee would be to act as a central reference point, it is likely the committee would meet frequently either to evaluate guidance sent to it or to consider proposals. Equally, it is highly desirable that the national ethical research committee is a compact body. For this reason, it is generally agreed that members of the national ethical research committee should be very senior and experienced people of distinction in their field. The suggested membership is as follows:

1 chairman nominated by the General Medical Council;
2 lay members nominated by the Secretary of State for Health and Social Security;
2 nominated by the Conference of Medical Royal Colleges and their Faculties;
1/2 nominated by Councils such as MRC (to be nominated in consultation with each other so that all relevant fields are represented);
1 nominated the Royal College of Nursing;
1 nominated by the Council for Professions Supplementary to Medicine;
1 nominated by the ABPI (in consultation with other groups in the pharmaceutical industry).

In addition, the national ethical research committee should have a panel of referees who would be nominated by the relevant professional group. It would be a requirement for the national ethical research committee to contact the appropriate referees.

It is thought undesirable for work to be undertaken by correspondence unless absolutely necessary as this places the lay members at an unfair disadvantage. They are already acting in areas where they are highly unlikely to have the same degree of scientific knowledge as others on the committee and should be given the opportunity to question and explore fully any aspects of a research proposal which cause them concern.

Funding

It is very important for the national ethical research committee to be seen to be independent. The responsibility of funding this should be with the government.

Bibliography

Abortion, contraception and sterilisation

Abortion Act 1967. Chapter 87. *London: HMSO, 1967.*

BMA Committee on Therapeutic Abortion. Indications for termination of pregnancy. *Brit Med J 1968; i: 171–5.*

Department of Health and Social Security. The use of fetuses and fetal material for research. Report of the Advisory Group. *London: HMSO, 1972.* (Peel Report).

Committee on the Working of the Abortion Act. Report. Vol I-III. *London: HMSO, 1974.* (Lane report) (Cmnd 5579-I, 5579-II).

Seller M. Congenital abnormalities and selective abortions. *J Med Ethics 1976; 2: 138–41.*

Tunkel V. Abortion: how early, how late, and how legal? *Brit Med J 1979, ii: 253–6.*

Gardner R F. The ethics of abortion. *Practitioner 1979; 223: 244–8.*

Duncan S L B. Ethical problems in advising contraception and sterilisation. *Practitioner 1979; 223: 237–42.*

Anonymous. Late consequences of abortion. (Leader) *Brit Med J 1981; 282: 1564.*

Consent to treatment

Garnham J C. Some observations on informed consent in non-therapeutic research. *J Med Ethics 1975; 1: 138–45.*

Anonymous. Valid parental consent. *Lancet 1977; i: 1346–7.*

Clothier C M. The law and the juvenile donor. *Lancet 1977; i: 1356–7.*

Skegg P D G. English law relating to experimentation on children. *Lancet 1977; ii: 754–5.*

Anonymous. Human experimentation: human rights. *J Med Ethics 1978; ii: 1352.*

Vere D. Testing new drugs: the human volunteer. *J Med Ethics 1978; 4: 81–3.*

Anonymous. Consent to treatment. *Brit Med J 1979; i: 1091–2.*

Dunstan G R, Seller M J. Consent in medicine: convergence and divergence in tradition. *London: King's Fund Centre, 1983.*

Kirby M D. Informed consent: what does it mean? *J Med Ethics 1983; 9: 69–75.*

Genetics

Ellis H L. Parental involvement in the decision to treat spina bifida cystica. *Brit Med J 1974; i: 369–72.*

Newcastle Regional Hospital Board Working Party. Ethics of selective treatment of spina bifida. Report. *Lancet 1975; i:85–8.*

Arnold A, Moseley R. Ethical issues arising from human genetics. *J Med Ethics 1976; 2: 12–17.*

Health and Safety Commission. Genetic manipulation, regulations and guidance notes. *London, HMSO, 1978.*

Ethics Advisory Board. Health, education and welfare support of research involving human in vitro fertilization and embryo transfer – report and conclusions. *Washington: US Government Printing Office, 1979. (017-040-00453-2).*

Harris J. Ethical problems in the management of some severely handicapped children. *J Med Ethics 1981; 7: 117–24.*

Seller M J. Ethical aspects of genetic counselling. *J Med Ethics 1982; 8: 185–8.*

British Medical Association. Interim report on human in-vitro fertilisation and embryo replacement and transfer. Report of Working Group on In-Vitro Fertilisation. Annual Report of Council 1983, Appendix VI, *Brit Med J 1983; 286: 1594–5.*

Industrial action

Anonymous. Strikes in the National Health Service. *J Med Ethics 1977; 3: 55.*

Dworkin G. Strikes and the National Health Service: some legal and ethical issues. Commentary by P Zacharias. *J Med Ethics 1977; 3: 76–82.*

Royal College of Nursing. Code of professional conduct: a discussion document. *J Med Ethics 1977; 3: 115–23.*

Conference of Royal Medical Colleges of UK and BMA, Joint Working Party. Discussion document on ethical responsibilities of doctors practising in the National Health Service. *Brit Med J 1977; i: 157–9.*

Insemination, artificial

British Medical Association. Report of Panel on Human Artificial Insemination. Board of Science and Education. Annual Report of Council 1972, Appendix V. *Brit Med J 1973; ii: 3–5.*

Harrison R F, Wynne Williams G. Human artificial insemination. *Brit J Hosp Med 1973; 9: 760–2.*

Cusine D J. AID and the law. *J Med Ethics 1975; l: 39–41.*

Cusine D J. Medico-legal aspects of AID. *IPPF Medical Bulletin 1979; 13: 1–2.*

Anonymous. Artificial insemination for all. *Brit Med J 1979; ii: 458.*

British Medical Association, ARM. Legitimacy for AID children. *Brit Med J 1979; ii: 70.*

Professional confidence

Home Office. Report of the Committee on Privacy. *London: HMSO, 1972.* (Younger report) (Cmnd 5012).

World Medical Association. Computers and confidentiality in medicine. *Brit Med J 1973; ii: 290–3.*

Barber B, Cohen R D, Kenny D J, Rowson J, Scholes M. Some problems of confidentiality in medical computing. *J Med Ethics 1976; 2: 71–3.*

Home Office. Report of the Committee on Data Protection. *London: HMSO, 1978.* (Lindop report) (Cmnd 7341).

Diamond B. Medical confidentiality and the law. *World Medicine 1979; 14: 63–4.*

Thompson I E. The nature of confidentiality. *J Med Ethics 1979; 5: 57–64.*

Pheby F H. Changing practice on confidentiality: a cause for concern. *J Med Ethics 1982; 8: 12–24.*

Terminal illness and death

British Medical Association. The problem of euthanasia. Report of a Special Panel of the Board of Science and Education. *London: BMA, 1971.*

Nicholson R. Should the patient be allowed to die? *J Med Ethics 1975; 1: 5–9.*

Campbell A G M. Moral dilemmas in the care of the dying. *Mimms Magazine 1978; 2: 623–9.*

Campbell A G M, Duff R S. Deciding the care of severely malformed or dying infants. *J Med Ethics 1979; 5: 65–7.*

Lawton, Lord Justice. Mercy killing: the judicial dilemma. *J Royal Soc Med 1979; 72: 46–1.*

Sweet T. Good or bad law. *J Royal Soc Med 1979; 72: 461–4.*

Rhoades J D J. The right to die and the chance to live. *J Med Ethics 1980; 6: 53–4.*

Havard J D J. The legal threat to medicine. *Brit Med J 1982; 284: 612–3.*

Law Reform Commission of Canada. Euthanasia, aiding suicide and cessation of treatment. Report. *Ottawa: Government Catalogue J31-40, 1983.*

British Medical Association. Euthanasia. Report of the Working Party on Euthanasia. *London: BMA, 1988.*

Transplantation

Jenet B. The donor doctor's dilemma: observations on the recognition and management of brain death. *J Med Ethics 1975; 1: 63–6.*

Knight B. Law and ethics in transplantation. *Practitioner 1976; 216: 471–4.*

Anonymous. Coroners and transplants. *Brit Med J 1977; i: 1418.*

Kennedy I. The donation and transplantation of kidneys: should the law be changed? *J Med Ethics 1979; 5: 13–21.*

Sells R A. Live organs from dead people. *J Royal Soc Med 1979; 72: 109–17.*

Department of Health and Social Security. Cadaveric organs for transplantation. A code of practice, including the diagnosis of brain death, drawn up and revised by a Working Party on behalf of the Health Departments of Great Britain and Northern Ireland. *London: HMSO, 1983.*

General

Ramsey P. The patient as person. *New Haven and London: Yale University Press, 1970.*

Taylor J Leahy. The doctor and the law. *London: Pitman Medical and Scientific Publishing Co Ltd, 1970.*

Veatch R M. Case studies and medical ethics. *Cambridge Mass: Harvard University Press, 1977.*

Duncan A S, Dunstan G R, Wellbourn R B. Dictionary of Medical Ethics. *London: Darton, Longman and Todd, 1981.*

Gillon R. The function of criticism. *Brit Med J 1981; 283: 1633–9.*

Sieghart P. Professional ethics – for whose benefit? *J Med Ethics 1982; 8: 25–32.*

British Medical Association. The occupational physician. *London: BMA, 1982.*

Association of British Pharmaceutical Industries. Data sheet compendium 1983–84. *London: Datapharm Publications, 1983.*

General Medical Council. Professional conduct and discipline: fitness to practise. *London: GMC, 1983.*

Mason J K, McCall R A. Law and medical ethics. *London: Butterworths, 1983.*

British Medical Association. The Handbook of Medical Ethics. *London: BMA, 1984.*

British Medical Association. Selection of Casualties For Treatment After Nuclear Attack. Discussion document. Board of Science and Education, *London, 1988.*

Index